No Gym Go Slim

"Easily learn and understand how the body works
to help you take control of your weight and health."

"Finally gain the knowledge
to truly become healthier for the rest of your life."

"Be healthy for today and tomorrow!"

By: Dr. Richard L. Sheppard

No Gym Go Slim

Written by Dr. Richard L. Sheppard

ISBN: 1490312692
ISBN-13: 9781490312699

Table of Contents

acknowledgements: I have been reading and studying health for nearly 20 years. I have read countless studies, books and purchased many programs myself. This includes all the textbooks of anatomy, physiology and biochemistry during my Chiropractic education.

I recognize that I may fail at giving credit to all of those that inspire me or even to those I have used as some references in my book. I did my best to acknowledge where a reference has come from.

The many books, websites, publications and newsletters that I have read and continue to do so, are part of the process of continual learning, expanding and growing as a person, a doctor and a learner.

I recommend the following sources:

Dr. Mercola of Mercola.com

Mike Adams, the Health Ranger @ Naturalnews.com.

Book: *Burn the Fat, Feed the Muscle* by Tom Venuto

The company Precision Nutrition @ Precisionnutrition.com

Of course my book would not be possible without my loving wife, Carrie. She continues to be my biggest supporter and best friend for nearly 30 years. Without her love and inspiration, this book and any accomplishments in my life would not be possible.

please read: Before you start any new exercise program or make any changes with your nutritional plan, it is always good to have a discussion with your health care provider about implementing any changes.

introduction: Welcome and thank you for purchasing my book called *No Gym Go Slim*. Let me introduce myself. My name is Dr. Richard Sheppard. I am a practicing Doctor of Chiropractic and have been doing so for over 16 years. I have owned and operated eight clinics in three different states. I am asked on a daily basis from my patients to help them with weight loss.

The first question that I ask anyone who wants to lose weight, is how committed are you to losing weight? I am going to tell you immediately in the *Introduction* of this book, that weight loss is extremely easy. Yes it is. It takes two things -- a little discipline and some time. I remind my patients that next year is coming, and so is next summer, and another year. It is your future, be there healthy.

The body is a little more complex than simply counting calories. You will learn that calorie reduction will work for a short period of time, but then your body will start using bone and muscle tissue as fuel. That is why crash dieters always end up gaining more weight back than when they started. This book is based on science, not fads.

Gaining weight did not occur over the

period of a week or two, or a month or two. It takes months and months, and frankly years and years, of mismanagement of food and lifestyle choices to cause weight gain and store fat. As you are reading this book, it is quite clear that I do not know you, your age, your weight, your medical history, or anything about you. But what I do know is that, with the exception of a severe medical condition, you still can lose weight. Please understand that when I talk about weight loss, we are not talking about losing a few pounds on the scale, or even many pounds on the scale for that matter. I am talking about burning fat, making your body more lean and muscular, which will allow for a healthier and happier life. Bathroom scales serve one purpose, which I will mention later.

Let us discuss some numbers. At the time I am writing this book, there are currently approximately 7 billion people in the world. Nearly 1.6 billion are overweight. In the United States there are over 300 million people -- 200 million people are considered overweight, with 100 million of those people classified as obese. The cost of being overweight and/or obese is about $150 billion a year in related costs, health-care costs and products, pills, potions, and lotions for losing weight.

You can lose weight by dieting, exercising, pills, supplements, or risky surgery. The facts are only about 10% of the country exercise regularly. I will tell you from my observations and experiences, even the people that go and exercise and make an effort -- most of them are wasting their time. They will never lose any weight, they will not change their body composition. Certainly by getting off your butt and walking on a treadmill or using the exercise bike and sweating with or without a friend offers benefits, but a lot of people never really change their bodies. There is a reason why when everybody gets a new calendar they try and then struggle for about four, five, or six weeks and then quit. The average person that wants to lose weight has tried four times in one year.

Do you want to join one of the big corporate weight loss chains? They take $3 billion out of American consumer's pockets each year with little success. Want to try diet pills? That is also a $3 billion per year market. Do you honestly think by taking some pill advertised by the Kardashians that you would look like them with little to no effort? The answer to that question is no. In this book I will offer a few specific supplements that your body needs. They are requirements for your body and overall health. I will also inform you that, if you truly want to lose weight, you are going to have to avoid something that you are eating or drinking right now. Here is something I tell my patients -- I want you to memorize this phrase, "nothing tastes as good as thin and fit feels".

How this book will apply to the rest of your life is like treating your body like a corporation. You are the CEO in charge of your corporation -- the CEO of your body. How well you effectively manage your corporation (body) will dictate if you are going to turn a profit, breakeven, or suffer a loss. This is a nice analogy, but many of you are mismanaging your corporation and ultimately ruining your health. I can hear Donald Trump telling you, "You're Fired!"

How many of you have tried to lose weight and failed, tried again and failed, maybe a third time and failed, maybe for the 20th time and failed? When you base your efforts on fads, or what your brother's cousin's neighbor's friend tried and worked for them, may surely not work for you. There are copious amounts of books out there: Atkins, Zone Diet, The Reverse Diet, Baby Food Diet (thanks Jennifer Aniston), Blood Type Diet, Caveman Diet, Grapefruit 45, Cabbage Soup, and many other products that you may have tried.

My book is called *No Gym Go Slim*. I say you do not have to work out hours and hours to lose weight. There is a saying for those of you that go to the gym and want to have a flat stomach that "abs are made in the gym", but actually "abs are made in the kitchen". Another phrase I want you to memorize, and I mean print it out or write it on a postcard or post-it note and look at it every day and remind yourself of, is this – "it's not what you do all the time, it's what you do most of the time that matters".

Now, let me be clear, even though my book is called No Gym Go Slim, I have a chapter in here if you want to exercise. You can make your weight loss more efficient for fat burning and putting on lean muscle. However, you need to understand the importance of that as you read my book, that that chapter is about fat burning and muscle gain. A joke I tell to my patients that ask me what I do for workouts is: on Monday I work out my chest and back, Wednesday I do arms and shoulders, and Friday it is pizza and chicken wings. The joke is that I do not do that every Friday, but if I am conscious of the fact that I take care of my body Monday through Friday, surely I can enjoy the pleasures of my favorite foods.

As a Doctor of Chiropractic, there are some patients that many times I will not see for six months or maybe even a year. Now, this is not a book about my Chiropractic practice, but, I have a wellness practice which means I see people once or twice a month when they are well, to stay that way -- wow what a concept! My biggest observation over the past 15 years is seeing how fast health can take a turn. I have seen it go both ways. I have seen people, which I consider the upright dead. Meaning they simply have not fallen over yet. However, with the proper care and nutrition, they can turn into really healthy individuals. Most of the time, when I have not seen somebody for six months to a year, it is not, "wow, you look great I can't believe it!", it is more like, "oh my gosh, what happened to you?"

There is nothing we can do about getting older. I tell this to my friends all the time. I say, I do not have a fear of getting older, but I am petrified of being old. Yet I see it every day in my practice. Most of what I see is what occurs in this country with our health and our weight. Most of the time conditions can be prevented, fixed, and reversed. However, the only person that is preventing this from happening is <u>you</u> -- <u>you</u> get in your own way.

There were many titles that I rolled around in my head for this book. I thought of -- *One Life One Body, It's Your Health, In Your Health* -- I even considered, *It's Your Health Why Don't You Care More*. My book is based on science and science alone. When you understand how the body functions, it is then that you can fix it and help it. In addition to the science, I am going to give you some background information. We are going to set up a knowledge foundation so that you understand the "what" and the "why". The word "doctor" means "teacher". My job is to educate and hopefully motivate. I do not know you personally, but there are going to be times that you are reading this book and feel that I am talking to you directly. Sometimes, you are going to feel that I am so in your face, and who is Dr. Sheppard to say that to me. Frankly, some of you need that. You bought this book with a want and a need to lose weight.

So many people quit way too soon, stop way too soon, and do not wait long enough for the results. If you learn anything from my book and are successful, it will motivate you to keep going. Fads, pills, and surgeries are the norm these days. But, how do you really fix things? You do it with science, with principles, and with nature. I promise you, by the time I finish writing this book and get it out there, another fad will be sold that millions of you will try.

I have asked my patients, if they can only have one option in relation to their health, and their choices are: exercise, chiropractic, or nutrition (of course there are many things to allow you to become healthier), but if you could only choose one, I am telling you, the correct answer is nutrition.

I enjoy exercising. I completed the home program called P90X, and I have done five marathons. I have worked out my entire life because I enjoy it. When I need or want to make a change in my body and my health, it is not the exercise; it is the nutritional changes that move me forward.

In this book you are going to learn what to avoid and what to eat. You will no longer feed your body you will fuel your body. You will eat to live, not live to eat. You will lose weight as a normal body process. You will no longer be overfed and undernourished. You will become healthier – period. You will add quantity and quality to your life. Life is an adventure of learning and experiencing. Let us enjoy and embrace the journey. Be well for today and tomorrow.

Chapter 1

Knowledge is Power

Actually, the title of the chapter is wrong. Knowledge is not power. The <u>application</u> of knowledge is power. We all know that smoking is bad for us, dangerous, and even addictive, but how many still choose to smoke? It is the application of knowledge that is truly powerful.

This chapter, as well as many in this book, is designed to educate and hopefully motivate. I claim not to be Tony Robbins, but I do claim to possess knowledge of the human body, anatomy, physiology, and a basic foundational understanding of nutrition. I will do my best to teach the fundamentals of health and nutrition. The side effect will be your more efficient, fat-burning machine of a body.

If you are reading this book, it means you are in a position in your life right now that you have decided that it is time to lose weight and become healthier. That is the first step. With that first step, is the word "honest". You must be honest with yourself and understand that your weight gain, being out of shape, or not being as healthy as you could be, did not occur overnight. It takes time to gain weight. Sure, if you went ahead and weighed yourself on a Monday and ate junk all week, there is a chance you could gain a few pounds during that week. What I am talking about is months and months and years and years of mismanagement of your health and nutrition.

In this book, the bathroom scale is not something that we are going to rely on. Try and imagine, for example, if you weighed a certain amount of pounds and you lost 10 pounds of fat, but replaced it with 10 pounds of muscle. Clearly the scale would read exactly the same weight, but your appearance and physique would be remarkably better.

I do not mind using a bathroom scale to check for initial weight loss, or to see how certain foods react with our body by holding onto water, etc. Here is a great trick to train your brain to lose weight with the scale. I want you to print out the weight you want to be at, regardless of where you are now. Then tape it over the window on the scale. Every morning, I want you to close your eyes, step on the scale and tell yourself, "every day, in every way, I am becoming lean and healthier". Then, look down and open your eyes and see your weight. The more you do this exercise, the more your brain will believe it. Eventually, your mind will start moving you towards that goal. The book, Think and Grow Rich, by Napoleon Hill, is a great way to re-program your brain to think better thoughts.

If we take a look at the weight loss and exercise fitness industry, it is over $30 billion per year. If these big corporate chains had such tremendous success or the weight loss products were so successful in helping people lose weight, there would not be a need for new products. There would not be any more new books. Each and every year there is a new book that tells you – do not eat that, do this, or do that. While some of them offer some good advice, others are just fads.

Now, in my book, you are going to get the knowledge and then you will decide what to do with it. I would say that, right now, losing weight is easy. It may be the easiest thing I could have you do. But, you must understand that the weight did not go on overnight and it will not leave overnight. If you are someone who has bought into the commercial that says, "lose 30 pounds in 30 days", well, you frankly got snookered.

My book, and the information that you are going to learn, is science. We are not trying to "make weight" for the high school wrestling team before the big match. I am not talking about losing water so the scale goes down or to see if you fit into a certain size jeans. I am talking about long-term weight loss -- more lean muscle, less body fat, and a healthier you -- not for today and tomorrow, but for the rest of your life.

You are going to learn about the macronutrients. There are three macronutrients: Proteins, carbohydrates, and fats. Proteins are necessary for lean muscle and to keep your body functioning. Carbohydrates (carbs) are also necessary. But carbs have to be the correct kind. It does not necessarily mean you have to cut out bread and pasta from your life. There are strategies to allow you to actually have more good tasting carbs and not allow your body to have a negative response to them. Some of the responses that the body has with certain nutrition are things you heard of, but may not fully understand. Things such as the glycemic index of foods. You may have heard of that before but do not understand what it means. There is also something called the glycemic load, which is more important than the glycemic index. I will be talking about the difference between them. The last of the macronutrients is fats. Fat gets a bad rap. Most people do not understand that fats are very necessary. We need fats, good fats, in our diet. There is a whole section of this book devoted to fats, and I am going to tell you, that if you try to cut out fat from your diet with all these products in the market today being no fat, low fat and fat-free, what you will get is more fat on you. I say that when you find a product in the store that says fat-free, that means the fat you do not have to pay for.

The human body is the most incredible machine ever invented. It is a self-regulating and self-healing organism. You want to talk about miracles? It is a miracle that someone can start their day with a whole bunch of crappy food and the body will take some of it and do its best to convert it to energy and skin cells or red blood cells and repair itself. That is a miracle!

If you are looking for a book that is going to spoon feed you, this may not be for you. You may actually have to do a little homework and do a small amount of testing to find out what works for you. When I talk about this book also being motivating, I am serious about that.

Answer this question for me; what is the difference between you and me? What is the difference between someone who lost weight and someone that did not? What is the difference of 20 successful people and that one not successful person? Outside of the specific answer, those answers are not very much different.

I would tell you that as a Chiropractor in my own office, other Chiropractors, and my Chiropractic friends constantly contact me and ask me what I would do here and how are you doing this. I tell them, the difference between your business and my business, is the fact that you are always trying to hit a home run when I try to get a lot of base hits and an occasional double. What that means, is that your typical Chiropractor wants to do one advertisement and get 50 new patients. I do not know one way to get 50 new patients, but I know 50 ways to get one new patient. Apply that to weight loss. If you need to lose 20, 30, 40, 50 pounds or more, I am sure you want it overnight. You want to run out and get gastric bypass and liposuction or take a magic pill, potion, or lotion. You surely can do those things, but, if you do not change your basics, you will still struggle with your health and your weight regardless of the short cut.

I would rather have you tweak your lifestyle in small increments which allows for a greater success and a greater change overall. Please learn from this book, starting with the very next chapter. For example, do you eat breakfast or do you skip it? I will tell you as a general rule, and there are always exceptions to the rule, as I talked about smoking earlier. Sure there is that one person out there who is 80 years old, in great health, but has smoked since he was 15. Is that the rule or the exception? So as a general rule, if you are skipping breakfast in the morning, your chances of being overweight are much greater than somebody who eats breakfast.

In this chapter I say knowledge is power. Again it is the application of knowledge that is power. I went through the New Year's resolutions with my friends. I saw one of them bought a $200 juicer. He spent the first 7 to 10 days of the New Year juicing and dropped 20 pounds. Fast-forward to today (about 30 days later) and this person is 25 pounds heavier. You cannot just go ahead and make these radical extreme changes in your life and expect to stick with it or do something that you just cannot do every day. That type of person is right now waiting for the next fad. Life is not a spectator sport. I want to get in the game. I want to play.

Take a baby learning to walk. They fall down, try again, fall down again, and fall, fall and fall. How many times does your baby need to fall before you, as a parent, say, well they just cannot do it, they are never going to learn to walk. You would not do that. You know they are going to walk, they want to walk, they will not stop until they do. So the question is, why don't you have that kind of determination and desire for your weight loss?

We are all products of our environment. What does that mean? It means simply if your parents go to church every Sunday, then you, as a child, go to church every Sunday. If your family growing up is active, then you are active. If you like to cook and eat dinner at the table with the T.V. off, then that is probably what you will do with your children. Today's world has got so fast and instant, we forgot the basics. Please understand that I am not asking you to eat next to nothing, with things that do not taste good, and never enjoy anything about food ever again. Hey, I was born and raised in Chicago, and Chicago has the best pizza. Trust me, when I visit Chicago, I am eating pizza.

Remember what I said, "it's not what you do all the time, it's what you do most of the time that matters". You will have times that you are really happy and want to have fun and eat and drink. You could have a really bad day and want some comfort food. There is nothing wrong with that. But, if you apply some of the basic principles, and the things you will learn here, and, have a little discipline, you will be so surprised at your results.

I want to tell you of a study that was done regarding the power of your mind. The fact that you are reading this book means you are taking the first step towards weight loss. Do not read this book just to read this book. I want you to get organized. I want you to set goals for yourself. I want you to set small goals and one huge goal. For example, your first goal might be to lose 10 pounds. Your second goal may be to lose an additional 5 to 10 pounds. Your huge goal may be to get down to a size four and lose 75 pounds. If you shoot for the stars and only hit the moon, you will be doing really well.

When I talked about the scale, I am not overly concerned with just weight loss in pounds. I am more concerned that you transform your body of burning the fat while creating more lean muscle and losing inches. Now, if you have a goal of losing 10 pounds, you should also do some measurements of your waist, hips, arms, etc.

Here is a goal for you and your bathroom scale that I previously talked about. I have personally done this and I swear to you it works. I want you to go to a store and buy the cheapest bathroom scale they have. The one I have has the small little window, spring-loaded, and not that accurate. Forget the digital scales or the ones that measure body fat. So, I printed out in big bold black numbers the weight I wanted to be. I taped this number on the scale window. Every morning I would get up and would say the following: "every day, in every way, I'm getting better and better". Then I would walk to my bathroom scale, take a deep breath in and out, stand on the scale, feel the pressure of the scale, hear my spring-loaded scale move back and forth, and look down at the numbers. You start convincing yourself of the weight you want to be. When you train your conscious brain to believe it, your subconscious brain will take over and lead to activities necessary to obtain that goal.

There was an experiment done on this and it has been repeated multiple times. They took a group of people and divided them into three groups. And let us say there were 100 people in each group for a total 300 people. So, for the experiment, they all went to the local gym and they all shot a number of free throws on the basketball court. Each group then had a percentage of free throws made. The first group, after the percentage was determined, was sent home and told not to shoot any free throws and come back in a month. The second group was told to come to the gym several days a week and practice shooting free throws. The third group was told not to go to the gym, but come to the classroom several days a week. The group in the classroom would spend time with their eyes closed visualizing standing at the free-throw line bouncing the ball, aiming, shooting the ball, and seeing the ball go in the basket.

At the end of four weeks, all the groups returned back to shoot free throws again. The group that did not practice, came back and shot free throws, did statistically about the same they did at the beginning. The second group that went to the gym three days a week to practice the free throws, all improved as a group. Practice does make perfect. The third group who spent their time in class visualizing making the free throws all improved! In fact, they improved almost as well as the group that physically practiced shooting free throws.

These kinds of studies, experiments, and books work time and time again. Other examples are the movie *The Secret* and the book by Napoleon Hill, *Think and Grow Rich*, which states, "what the mind can conceive and believe the body can achieve".

Before I elected to become a Chiropractor, I had no idea what I wanted to do for a career. I remember being 18 years old, out of high school, going to community college and driving around really nice neighborhoods, looking at these beautiful houses. Now, this is a time before the Internet, but I grabbed a flyer for this house that was for sale, which I thought was the most beautiful house ever. It was not the biggest house on the block, but it was what I wanted. I had that picture in a folder for years. Then I decided to become a Chiropractor, got through school, passed Boards, and started my own practice. Eventually, I was able to save enough money to build a house. When my house was built and when I moved in, I found that picture of my dream house that I had looked at ten years earlier. Guess what? The house that I built was almost identical in appearance to that house that I visualized.

So let us understand that weight loss is simply a time factor. If you put more time, energy, and effort into your weight-loss, it will work much faster. If you do not give it as much time and attention, it will take a really long time for you. Remember, where attention goes, energy flows. If you understand that health and healing and weight loss is not linear, it is not a straight line. There are bumps along the way. You may lose weight. You may lose 5 or 10 pounds, put on three pounds, lose three or four pounds, and again put three pounds on. The point is, if you stay focused and dedicated, to the best of your ability, you will 100%, guaranteed, lose weight.

As I said before, I will offer in this book a chapter on exercise. I will, however, offer it in a way that you could exercise less with more benefits. I promise you that there are things that you are eating right now that you think are okay to eat, or are even good for you, that are completely blocking you from losing weight.

I will also explain to you why these large corporate chains' percentage of success is so low, and it will shock you. Remember most diets fail. Most diets start on Monday and end on Friday. Most diets start at the beginning of the year and end by Valentine's Day. Do not allow that to happen to you. There is a wonderful home workout DVD program that you have all heard of, called P90X. One of the things that Tony Horton, the creator of P90X, says is to "keep pushing play". I want you to keep focused. Because you know what, summer is coming and so is 2014. You cannot stop it, but what you can do is be ready for it. It is your future, be there healthy.

To summarize this chapter, it is the <u>application</u> of knowledge that is power. Empower yourself and start right now thinking positive thoughts. Start the journey for YOU. Of course you can do it. If I paid you $1 million to lose weight, could you? YES! So take away the million dollars and the answer is still YES. Start with small goals and at least one large goal. Write them down. Put them on your desktop on your computer and even print it out for your car. Every day I read my goals. People that write their goals down accomplish them approximately 85% more often.

In the next chapter I am going to discuss proteins, carbs, and fats. We were all taught about calories, or at least we think we know what they are. I will tell you right now that calories in and calories out will work temporarily for weight loss. When I say temporarily, there are some really great apps for your smart phone or your computer -- like *My Fitness Pal*. That is a great app, but it is based on calories in and calories out. I will talk about why that will work temporarily and not for long-term. In this book I do not ask you to count calories, I am not asking you to measure food, nor will I ask you to starve yourself. I am going to ask you to discipline yourself and eat a little bit slower and smarter. If you can, then you can become healthier and lose weight.

Chapter 2

The How and The Why

This should be a pretty easy question to ask yourself -- why are you overweight? Answer: I eat too much, I eat the wrong stuff, I do not exercise, it is in my genes. Some of those statements may have some truth in them, but most of the time they are more excuses. So right now ask yourself, do you want reasons or results?

At the time I am writing this chapter, I am 43 years old. I feel like I am 23, and hopefully look less than 43. The interesting thing about the human body is that it changes as we get older. Yes, we know that. But, even our chemistry changes. We are not the same person we were 10 years ago, 20 years ago, or 30 years ago. Not even last year! Our body needs different nutrition than it did when we were younger. So it does not matter how old you are, your athletic background, or your past health history. What matters is, what are you going to do today to become healthier and lose weight?

I was the guy at the gym that you do not want to be next to on the treadmill. I would be on it longer than you, and I would sweat like nobody's business. Funny thing about that, I have completed five marathons and with all my running and cardio training, I still did not lose that much weight. I am not telling you not to exercise. I will, however, tell you, at the end of this book, how to make exercise more efficient so you do two things: burn fat and produce lean muscle via growth hormone release. Those two things, less fat and more lean muscle, will help you with your longevity. There is nothing wrong with taking a walk around the neighborhood after dinner. It certainly is better than sitting on the couch and watching TV. Getting some fresh air, some movement, raising the body temperature, increasing circulation, talking with a friend or family member is all great for stress reduction and offers some health benefits. But, I am going to tell you that you will not change your body fat or composition with just walking. I will be right, in the fact, that you will not lose much weight, if any, at all.

I am sitting, right now, writing this book, looking out my window after dinner, watching my neighbors walk. Great! I am glad to see people be more active. With the internet and cell phones we are all becoming much more sedentary. But, I will tell you it is not our lifestyle only that is dictating our poor health. It is the garbage that we call food that we are using to feed our body versus fuel our body.

We are eating way too many processed foods, not enough lean protein, and consuming way too much sugar. We consume so much sugar in the United States that it is enough per person to kill a small horse. Ok, I do not know if that is true or not, but we simply consume too much sugar and sugar-like products. It is not so much what we consume, but also how it reacts with our body.

Take for example alcohol. If you have ever had a glass of wine, beer, or shots, you know there are different ways that the same amount of alcohol can affect you. If you skip lunch or skip dinner and wind up at happy hour to have a few drinks, you know that alcoholic beverage will affect you sooner, harder, and faster versus the person that had a big lunch and a big dinner.

Food is no different. <u>Skipping breakfast is mighty mistake #1</u>. Again it is not about counting calories. I mentioned that there are some wonderful programs for your smart phones or computer that will work for awhile. But it will have what is called the law of diminishing returns. It is just like medication that you may be taking. Medicine is pretty effective the first time you use it. For example, an injection for neck or back pain will typically work pretty well for anywhere from three to six months. Of course, it will not take care of the underlying problem, so then the pain returns, and if you receive a second injection you will feel pretty good for two months, maybe three months. By the third round of injections it can have a minimal effect or none at all. It is how the body works and how the body functions. Take somebody who drinks alcohol five days a week versus someone who does not drink that much, and compare the difference in the amount that they can consume without feeling the effects of alcohol.

Food is a drug. We have gotten so far away from nature that we have too many chemicals in our body, coupled with too little of the good stuff like healthy fats. Yes you read that correctly, I said fats. We do not eat enough of fats because we think we are going to get fat from fats.

Let me tell you my problem with calories in and calories out. Do you know how many calories it takes to burn one pound? The answer is 3,500 calories. That means if you burn 500 calories a day more than you take in, meaning you have a deficit of 500 calories per day times seven days per week, you will lose one pound. Take the 200-pound guy or gal that does this for 50 weeks out of the year. Therefore, they should weigh 150 pounds after one year, assuming break even the first two weeks. That is a very real possibility in a very real scenario. Now year two, this person again breaks even for the first two weeks, and then for the next 50 weeks of year two they do the same scenario. They create a one-pound deficit each week for 50 weeks. This is another 50 pounds. Apply this scenario after three years. Do you honestly think this person is going to weigh 100 pounds or even 50 pounds? The answer is no. Certainly we have skin, bones, organs, and fluid and that we are never going to lose that amount of weight. But, eventually, by restricting calories too much, and too often, your metabolism will slow down. Your body will always be in survival mode.

I am getting into things like metabolism, calories, fats, carbs, and proteins. What are all of these things? Let us talk about some of these definitions.

There are so many products advertised that claim that they can speed up your metabolism and burn fat while you sleep. So what is metabolism? Metabolism is defined as the set of chemical reactions that occur in the cells of a living organism. While it is true that people with a faster metabolism can burn more calories at rest, have lots of energy, and are typically lean with a low percentage of body fat.

If you think by using caffeine you will lose weight, I will strongly disagree with you. The last thing that anyone ever needs is caffeine. Yes millions of Americans start their day with a cup of coffee to jump-start themselves. Now, if it is not coffee, it is an energy drink like Red Bull, Monster, or 5-Hour Energy. By sucking down so much caffeine we wonder why we cannot sleep at night. Add terrible food choices, artificial stimulants, lack of exercise, and you have got a major problem – it is brewing. But we will solve that problem with some pills – NO! I do not recommend any kind of medication or stimulant to help you sleep or get moving in the morning – Never! Remember this, most medications should be temporary until the problem is fixed.

Coffee by itself is not altogether bad, but when you start adding milk and sugar or worse yet artificial sweeteners, you have started your day behind the 8-ball. You are already setting yourself up for failure. In the coming chapters of this book I will discuss this further.

Calories. Stop right now and answer this: what is a calorie? Do you know the answer? Most people answer that by saying it is something in food. Answer: wrong. A calorie is a unit of measure, just like pounds, and like Fahrenheit or Celsius – it is a ruler. A calorie is defined as the amount of energy required to raise one gram of water one degree Celsius. If you suck down 2,000 calories at lunch, it may require your body a long time to process all of that. By the way, 2000 calories at lunch is way too much. You should be surviving on 2000 calories per day, unless you are performing a ton of activities or exercise.

Proteins. One of the three macronutrients is protein. I hope you are getting adequate amounts of protein. Did you ever wonder why grandma and grandpa get old and frail? It is not just because they are getting older. Have you ever looked at your grandmother's diet? My grandmother would start her day with a cup of tea. Lunch would be some crackers with a cup of soup, and for dinner a piece of pie.

The point is, grandma and grandpa do not eat enough protein. Your muscles are protein. Your brain, your skin, and a tremendous amount of your body's functions require adequate amounts of protein.

Examples of proteins are things like beef, chicken, fish, pork, eggs, and dairy (I do not recommend dairy by the way) beans, etc. The daily minimum requirement of protein is figured out by taking your weight in pounds and multiplying it by, at least, a third. For example, when you see an actor get buff for a film, like Hugh Jackman for Wolverine in The X-Men movies, he ate a tremendous amount of protein to get his body ready for that film. That is just one calculation for a minimum amount of protein. If you weigh 200 pounds and your body fat is at 20% (40 pounds), then subtract that and you get a lean body weight of 160 pounds. Then, based on your activity level, if you are very active, you might take your lean body mass and multiply by .8 if you are doing no exercise. This, of course, is a good way if you know your percentage of body fat. The best way to determine your body fat is to go to your local gym and get measured with calipers. There are body fat scales that are somewhat accurate, but do error on the high side.

The point is, if you measured for one week all the food that you ate, all the drinks that you drank, and recorded all of this, and actually looked at all the calories, and also looked at the number of grams of protein, you will probably find out that you are eating too many calories and not eating enough protein.

Carbohydrates. There are good carbs and there are bad carbs. The bad carbs you should know because they are in some of your favorite foods: bread, milk, potatoes, cookies, spaghetti, soft drinks, pizza, etc. Are you hungry yet? Sounds yummy. Just do not do it with every meal. Rule to practice: If you have some fun food, or please call it a reward meal, just do not do it with the very next meal you have. It is better for your progress and overall health.

Good carbs, in the simplest definition, are unprocessed and are in their natural state or very close to it. In other words, man or machine has minimally altered them. Green vegetables should be your new best friends. They are the best carbs for your body. Good carbs will be high in fiber, have a low glycemic index, high in nutrients, and will have a greater thermic effect that will naturally improve metabolism and promote fat loss. A partial list of good carbs is whole vegetables, whole fruits, beans, legumes, nuts, seeds, and whole grains. Go ahead and Google a full list if you need to.

The problem with bad carbs is like the example of drinking alcohol on an empty stomach. The bad carbs create such an insulin response, which affects blood sugar, which promotes fat storage and obesity. Listen to me as I tell you that it is okay to have bad carbs once in a while. Remember, "it's not what you do all the time, it's what you do most the time that matters". I will also mention that there is a trick that will allow you to earn a few more yummy carbs in your life.

Many of you are going to need to reset your body to have it function a little bit better and more normal. Some of you are going to follow my recommendations and will struggle with some initial weight loss. I may recommend a very specific cleanse to kick start your liver, your gallbladder, or your colon. Not only would you benefit from doing this once or twice each year, but you will be surprised at how your body will respond and start burning fat. Too many of you are burning sugar instead of primarily fat. Do not misunderstand; we do need carbs as well. It is just that getting into fat storage is the main goal.

It is kind of like gas prices for your car. You decide that you are going to solve the $4.00 per gallon price problem by putting half gas and half water in your tank, thinking it will reduce your gas bill to $2.00 per gallon. How do you think your car engine would feel about that? The answer is not very well. This is the analogy of what you are doing to your body by feeding it versus fueling it most of the time.

Fats. People hear the word fat and run for the hills. I cannot eat any fat because that is what makes me fat. Nothing could be further from the truth. I am going to tell you this. If you do not eat fat, you are going to be fat. Of your meal choices, 20% to sometimes 30% needs to include fat.

I will recommend several things in this book that I feel are requirements. One is a <u>good quality</u> fish oil supplement. You may have to pay a few extra dollars to actually get quality. At the end of this book I will have several links to several companies that I highly recommend and use for my family, my patients, and myself. Not only by taking this supplement will you lose weight, but you will actually help your body with inflammation and you will probably have less overall joint pain. Omega-3 fatty acids are the main ingredient in fish oil. You must get them in your diet with fish, eggs, and/or supplements. I prefer a combination of the three. I hate fish, but I eat it at least once a week.

Eggs are a staple in my diet. Notice I did not say egg whites. How the yolk became such an evil enemy in this country I will never know. Actual I do know the reason. Late in the 1960s and early 1970s there were studies done about cholesterol and heart disease. While the other camps were saying no it is the carbs that are causing heart disease and clogging arteries. The cholesterol camp won, and to this day, the top drugs in this country being sold are statin drugs to lower cholesterol.

My professional advice to you is to never take a statin/cholesterol-lowering drug unless it is absolutely necessary. The only exception to that rule is if your family history has a triglyceride count that is off the charts. Ninety-five percent of the people will not have that. There are so many side effects to these drugs. If you choose to take them, you must add a CoQ10 supplement. Essentially cholesterol drugs are good for the pipes, and are not good for the pump. Therefore, protect the pump with CoQ10. We need cholesterol in our bodies. Among other things, it produces hormones.

Did you know that our bodies in the liver, your internal organs, and your muscle tissue produce cholesterol? Just about every cell in your body has cholesterol. It is the building block of most essential hormones in your body. This is not a book about cholesterol, but is a book on health. Every time I tell people to eat a tremendous amount of eggs (eggs are not dairy, they are poultry), I get into a cholesterol debate. I am telling you that, if you look at websites such as Naturalnews.com or Mercola.com, you will discover and learn the dangers of chronic use of cholesterol drugs, along with the need for enzyme CoQ10. These are my two favorite health websites.

A list of good fats can also be found with a Google search. They include, but are not limited to, olive oil, canola oil, sunflower oil, avocados, olives, peanuts, cashews, hazelnuts, peanut butter, walnuts, flaxseed oil, and tofu.

The bad fats include dairy products, butter, cheese, etc. I am going to tell you to avoid dairy like the plague. Milk and cheese are out. If you are drinking milk because you enjoy the taste, I get it. But, if you are drinking milk because you think it offers health benefits, you are dead wrong.

Later in this book we will discuss why milk belongs to a baby cow and not a human. If you can walk and talk you do not need milk.

The Omega 3-fatty acids again are essential to your diet. Which means your body needs them so it can consume and convert them into things like painkillers, muscle relaxers, anti-inflammatories, and anti-depression meds – all naturally. In fact, Omega 3-fatty acids are so important, when you look at the ratio of Omega 6 and Omega 9, there has to be a balance. When that balance gets disrupted, poor health follows. When the disruption of ratios is so extreme, you get into clinical depression, schizophrenia, and even suicide and violent behavior. I am not suggesting that all the violent crimes that occur in this world can be solved by a fish oil supplement. But, what I am suggesting is that it is a necessary component for your body to function correctly. It is the difference between high premium gasoline and the water/gasoline mixture that I talked about.

Later in this book I will be discussing goal setting, executing a plan, and rewarding yourself with a cheat meal, which I like to call a reward meal. In life, you will determine that when your WHY is big enough, you will figure out the HOW. Start thinking about WHY you want to lose weight. It does not have to be one reason. It can be a multiple of reasons. But, if your WHY is not big enough, your HOW will never happen.

Let me explain this with a good friend of mine. He works 60 hours per week and is not fond of his job. When he gets home or not working, he does not want to exercise. So this book is perfect for him. But based on the stress, he right now has thrown in the towel. Since he feels that exercise is the only way to lose weight and he has no extra time in his mind, then he just eats whatever he wants. He eats a lot and he eats fast. By the way, fast is never a good idea when eating. His WHY is not big enough.

To summarize this chapter, it is more than simply calories in and calories out. It is the effect that food has on us and what our habits have been. You cannot skip breakfast and lose weight. You cannot just lower the number on a scale and call yourself healthy. You must make better choices. You cannot just buy some magic pill that will burn the fat or rev the metabolism. This is a larger problem that took time to develop. It will take time to un-do. I tell my patients, be a patient – patient!

In the coming chapters I will talk more about things that you will need to avoid. We all know someone that has been lean and muscular their whole life and we wish we had a body like them. These people may do all the things I am going to tell you not to do. I want to be very positive in this book and I do not want to tell you things that you can do because it sounds negative. I am going to say to you that if you do not listen to these chapters, then I am positive -- positive that you will fail. Do not let that happen. If I tell you not to drink milk, then do not drink milk. Guess what, if you decide in 30 or 45 days you want a glass of milk, it will be there. Do not freak out about what you cannot do, just start visualizing how you are going to handle all of the com-pliments of "Wow!" and "What have you been doing? You look amazing!".

Health is a choice. Too many people are spending their time buying at-home products, gym memberships, and just spinning their wheels. Life is a journey not a destina-tion. Weight loss and becoming healthier is also a journey with a destination. It is your future, be there healthy.

Chapter 3

Sleep and Genes

This chapter may be the shortest chapter I am going to write. For myself, I am a bottom-line type of guy, you know, the meat and potatoes kind. You now know the "How and the Why", we do not need all the extra fluff associated with it.

When I mentioned that this chapter is about sleep, there are no gray areas. The bottom line is sleep is something that is required. Your body needs sleep or you run the great probability of being overweight and probably obese.

I have plenty of male patients in my practice. Now, the majority of guys will be all macho and talk about how they work 23 ½ hours a day, sleep 5 minutes a day, and are still going strong. Let the truth be told that if there is any group of my patients making sacrifices and getting less sleep, it is the women. Let us be honest, most men are just big babies anyway. This includes me. My wife is a stay-at-home mom and, frankly, I have seen her job, and I do not want it.

Did you ever wonder what happens when you sleep? This is a time that your body uses to recoup, repair, and recover, but mainly REPAIR. Sleep is the best time for your body to self-regulate and prepare for the next day. Think of what happens if your body does not get to rest and repair. You get things like fatigue and lethargy and even sickness and disease. Think about a machine: your car when in use, an air-conditioning unit, or even a treadmill at the gym. All of these machines do not necessarily run all the time. Sure these machines can probably run 24/7, but they also need a break to cool off and get repairs. Even my home treadmill's manual states that after a certain amount of use a break should be given.

Remember this. When you sleep your body dissolves 2 stress hormones that promote obesity. They are cortisol and epinephrine. Deprive your body of sleep and you will not be able to adequately remove these stress hormones.

When you start thinking of your body as a business that you own, operate, and manage, it is also a highly efficient machine that you are required to maintain. If you do, you will soon be on your way to a healthier and thinner you. If you do not, then expect being a typical American that becomes overweight and sick.

The human body is a self-healing, self-regulating machine as I have mentioned before. When you disrupt the normal function over a continuous period of time, the body will give you signs and clues to let you know. If you ignore them, and then cover up the symptoms by taking a pill or by drinking a bunch of caffeine- laden drinks that will get you through the day, then future problems will be coming. Just remember, caffeine, in my opinion, is a drug. A drug without a side effect is not a drug. Caffeine also is great as a pesticide and too much of it is considered toxic. You have to love "medical experts" who say you can have this certain amount and it is still considered safe. Really? How much diluted poison would you consume if it was considered safe? Poor health is an accumulation of toxicity.

So let us get technical. Sleep is an important modulator of neuro-endocrine function and glucose metabolism. Sleep loss has been shown to result in metabolic and endocrine alterations including decreased glucose tolerance, decreased insulin sensitivity, increased evening concentrations of cortisol, increased levels of ghrelin, decreased levels of leptin, and increased hunger and appetite.

Cortisol, as you may or may not have heard of, is essentially your stress hormone. If lack of sleep increases cortisol, the stress hormone, then be prepared to be overweight. Again, you cannot simply just take a supplement or pop a pill to try to self-regulate hormones like cortisol.

There is a law in regards to pills, supplements, vitamins, and medication that you may be taking. It is called the law of diminishing returns. What this means is, that many times, a continued use of a medication, stimulant, drug, etc. will, in fact, be diminished over time the more you use it. The example is someone who rarely drinks alcohol. One or two drinks and this person may feel the effects of alcohol. If this person becomes a heavy drinker, then it may take seven or eight drinks to have the same effects as previous.

This is why I do not recommend anyone buy into these ideas of hormone replacement therapy as a way to regulate your body. It is important that you regulate your body with proper diet and even exercise. Understand that our bodies at 10 years old, 20 years old, 30 years old, and even 50 years old are different. Do not make the assumption that as your hormones change, then you simply need to supplement those levels. You may not need the same amount as you age. Do not mess with Mother Nature.

One thing I mentioned before when I said let us get technical, that by not getting enough sleep, it actually hurts the ability of fat cells to respond to insulin efficiently. As we continue on in this book and I give you a lot of the foundational framework to become healthier and lose weight, the goal is, with proper nutrition, you will fuel your body and not just feed your body. When we do this long enough, over time, your body will then be able to self regulate and you will then lose weight.

Without proper sleep, here is another process that occurs. When the cells fail to respond to insulin, lipids (or fats) can spill out in the bloodstream and surrounding tissue. When this happens, this insulin resistance, known as metabolic syndrome, is often a precursor to Type II, also called Adult Onset Diabetes. This is a study that was recently done in the Annals of Internal Medicine. The study said that if you are cramming for a final exam or have a newborn in your house and getting four hours of sleep, it is not unusual. Yet after just four nights of reduced sleep, it is the equivalent of metabolically aging 10 to 20 years. The study involved seven thin young healthy people with an average age just under 24. What would that do to you in your 30s, 40s, or 50s?

Most people need between seven and nine hours of sleep per night. Sleep degradation has been shown to reduce attention, slow reaction times, and impair learning. In addition, routine and frequent sleep deprivation will slow metabolism. And what is the "solution" for slow metabolism -- drugs and caffeine. Frankly, these poor choices will further affect your health in a negative way.

More studies need to focus on the effects of say getting more sleep on the weekends to see if that will reverse or help with the long-term of Monday through Friday sleep deprivation. Do not think you can work five days a week with very little sleep and then just make it up on the weekends. The body just does not work like that.

The magic number of hours needed, in the studies that I have read regarding sleep, seems to be about six hours. People are different. Some can do fine with six hours sleep and some require eight hours of sleep. It seems that when you get less than six hours of sleep, you are not giving yourself an adequate amount of rest. Anything over nine hours seems to be too long as far as having prolonged benefits. In addition to all that I have mentioned so far, other studies reveal how signals from the brain which control appetite regulation are impacted by sleep deprivation were the hormone ghrelin, which increases appetite and leptin, tells you that you are done eating. Translation – you are overweight.

Now sleep and stress seem to go hand-in-hand. You may be overstressed and worried about finances, job, career, kids, etc. and that increased stress can cause weight gain and will also affect the way you sleep. The reverse is also true as well. If you are not getting enough sleep, that can affect your performance at work, school, and relationships.

I always tell my patients that your spine did not get this way overnight, unless there was an accident. Typically it took years to get that way. You can reverse so much in terms of your health. So, put your body in reverse and un-do while you re-do the new healthier you.

I will tell you that if you start eating better, you will start feeling better. Even though this book is called No Gym Go Slim, exercise is a great way to help you go to sleep. For example, if you have children that have difficulty sleeping at night, or if you have a puppy in your home, the way that you make the puppy sleep and you make sure your children crash at the end of the night is to make sure they burn all that energy during the day.

When you start eating better and allow your body to get back to a state of higher functioning, sleep will not be a problem. If you decide to exercise, cardio-type exercises are not a good idea right before bed. Cardio-type activities actually increase brain activity, are stimulating, and will keep you awake. Weight training, or resistance exercise, can do those things too, but are best served doing at the end of the day, which will fatigue your body and help you sleep.

If you are having trouble sleeping on a regular basis, or for a long period of time, I highly recommend that you take the time to find a good Chiropractor and start getting spinal adjustments. I cannot tell you how many of my patients have told me that since they began Chiropractic care, not only are they out of pain and have more energy, but they sleep so much better at night. It makes sense, from the simple standpoint, that if you have pains that are waking you up at night, Chiropractic care can eliminate those pains naturally and you will sleep better through the night. Chiropractic has also been shown to help regulate your body so that you are able to sleep.

Continuous lack of sleep can cause the following: Dramatically weakened immune system, accelerated tumor growth, increased risk of heart disease, pre-diabetes, increased stomach ulcers, impaired memory, constipation, increased depression, and a host of other disorders.

The bottom line is to do several things. First, try and set your schedule to go to bed at the same time every night. Second, try no T.V. in your bedroom or do not use it to fall sleep with. The illumination from the T.V. will stimulate areas of your brain and actually keep you awake. You need a very quiet, very dark room for optimal sleeping conditions. I have reached the point in my life where I do not even need an alarm clock to wake up. I wake up at the same time every day. I am a creature of habit. I am so used to waking at the same time every day, that my body is now conditioned to this lifestyle.

The following tips can help you improve your sleep and your health: Sleep in a completely dark space, keep the temperature around 70 degrees, no T.V., avoid loud alarms, do not use the snooze bar, do not change your sleep schedule, do not take long naps during the day, do not eat sugar at bedtime, and avoid coffee and caffeine.

Again, "it's not what you do all of the time, it's what you do most of the time that matters". Things are going to occur in your life where you have to get up earlier, or stay up late to finish a project, or go out one night and party too long, etc. Some of you may have a changing work schedule. The point is, if you are concerned with your weight, and more importantly your overall health and well being, do your best to set a schedule that allows for at least six hours of uninterrupted sleep each night.

Also, if you find time or have the ability, a 15 to 20 minute nap during the day can be very beneficial. It will not only give you an energy boost, but it will help you sleep at the end of the day as well.

Now, briefly I want to talk about genes and genetics. There are a lot of things we get from our parents: hair color, eye color, bone structure, height, etc. Many of my patients have just made the assumption that since their mom or dad are overweight, that they are just destined to be overweight also. And while there may be some truth to that, for the most part, it is not the genes that you have, but what occurs to them. I have several families in my practice right now. The mom, dad, son, and daughters are all overweight. This is not a genetic factor with this family. It is the fact that they all eat the wrong stuff and way too much of it. I also have a few teen-aged girls that essentially starve themselves to be thin, when in reality; by not eating they are creating the very problem they are trying to avoid.

Take, for example, women that are concerned with breast cancer. Breast cancer may run in the family, you may have that gene that makes you more likely to get breast cancer. However, I do not think the surgical removal of your breasts is the answer for protection of breast cancer. You personally may be more prone to something in your genes versus someone else, but that is not the whole story.

There is a branch of science called epigenetics. Epigenetics basically says that it is really not what is in your genes that matter. It is what we do that affects our genes that matters. We, frankly, can turn things off or on. The precise definition of epigenetics is the development and maintenance of an organism, which is orchestrated by a set of chemical reactions that switch parts of the genome often on at strategic times and locations. Epigenetics is the study of these reactions and the factors that influence them. Your genes will dynamically respond to the environment, toxins, and other factors, which activate chemicals, which regulate gene expression. Essentially, what you do can turn them off and on, for better or for worse, the ultimate DNA marriage.

I am sure I can get into a whole bunch of arguments about genes and genetics. I will use my wife as an example. All the women in my wife's family have wide hips. Wide hips are great for childbearing, but not so if she wants to wear those tiny jeans. Does that mean based on her genetics that she cannot be thin and slim? No. What it means is her bone structure may come in to play, but she still is able to be lean and have a low percentage of body fat. So do not be so concerned with your genes, it is what you do with those genes that matters. Yes there are plenty of people that won the genetic lottery and are lean, muscular, thin, and beautiful. I am not one of them. Darn it!

It is quite possible and highly probable that YOU can improve you. Remember, this thing called life is a journey not a destination. Enjoy the ride! Your only competition is with you. You vs. you! The winner is YOU!

To summarize this chapter – Do not be a macho man. Get a bare minimum of six hours of sleep per night. Try and go to sleep at the same time every night. Sleep in a completely dark room with as little noise as possible. Do not try and catch up on sleep over the weekend. And, short naps are a good thing.

Be well for today and tomorrow. It is your health!

Chapter 4

Protein

I know the title of this book is *No Gym Go Slim*, but I will say it several times, you can, of course, exercise and further improve your health and I would like you to. Despite the title of this book, I will have some tips and strategies at the end that will maximize your exercise returns if you do elect to exercise. Physical fitness is important.

The problem that most people run into is that their nutrition will fail them. If you look at the top causes of death in the United States, you see things like heart disease, cancer, obesity, and diabetes. These diseases, that are killing us, are all nutritional related. So many things that we do, that affect our health in a negative way, are because of our choices.

I have run five marathons, I have exercised and weight lifted. I have been a big fan of exercise my entire life. It is fun for me. It offers stress relief and health benefits. But, I will say it again, if you want to see your abs – they are made in the kitchen, not the gym. It is sad to me that I see people exercising at the gym and they do not lose a pound or change their body. They do not lose an inch. They do not add muscle to their body. Frankly, they are wasting their time.

So does that mean if you go to the gym and use a treadmill or do the elliptical that you are wasting your time? Answer: No! There are indirect benefits to exercise. Let us say you walk 30 minutes on a treadmill during your lunch hour and you do that with a coworker or a friend. You are moving around; hopefully you are sweating a little bit and increasing circulation. All of that has tremendous benefits indirectly. Directly, you are not working hard enough to burn fat, or stimulating a growth hormone release from your body, which will allow for more lean muscle. With that example, you will not experience a change with your physique if that is your goal.

It all comes down to nutrition. How many people have you seen at the mall or your neighborhood that walk? There is nothing wrong with walking and getting some fresh air, but these are the people that are typically overweight and do not lose weight.

As I write this chapter, we are getting close to New Year's resolution time. And while I applaud anybody that makes an effort for any goal in their life, New Year's resolutions are the worst for success. I never understood why it takes a brand-new calendar and a brand-new year to change your life. If you are reading this book and it is Tuesday and it is the middle of March are you going to wait for January 1st to make a change? Being a doctor, I am exposed to a lot of people. For nearly two decades of treating patients I have noticed patterns of personalities. I can pretty much tell within the first few minutes of meeting a new patient if they are going to be a good patient, have compliance, make a change, or truly care enough about their health to be proactive.

One of the reasons that people fail with weight loss as a New Year's resolution is a poor understanding of fitness and nutrition. Here is what happens. After all the holiday parties and all the holiday stress, life returns back to a normal routine. You decide that you are going to lose weight. You take your work schedule and/or your school schedule and/or your family schedule and your life that is already busy and loaded responsibilities, and then you add exercise to it. It is something that was not there before that you have now added to your schedule. When your motivation produces minimal to no results, and your life stress soars, something will get dropped. The first thing that you drop is typically the last thing that is added. That thing is exercise. Look, habits are hard to form and they are also hard to break. You have a routine that you like your coffee in the morning and you have your bagel or doughnut. Friday night you go out for dinner and Saturday night is this, and Sunday's football, etc. I get it and I fully understand. You will need to make a list of the reasons why you want be healthier and you want to lose weight. When your WHY is large enough, you will then determine the HOW.

I do go to the gym and I do exercise. The pattern at my gym is usually around mid-January to mid-February my gym is very crowded, with a lot of new faces, waiting to use the equipment and a lot of crowded locker rooms. Then, by about March 1st, it is all back to normal. I find that very sad for many reasons. You had all the drive and determination in the world a short time ago and now you did not get the results you wanted and already quit. That is demoralizing. Right back to your normal routine, things do not change, your life moves on and the next thing you know you are making another New Year's resolution, but now you are 10 or 15 pounds heavier. It does not have to be that way. Start with nutritional changes first and the rest will follow. It is not a lack of exercise that causes you to gain weight, it is the nutritional choices that you made and the effect they have on you.

Did I not say the title of this chapter is protein? I am going to talk about protein now. It is really important for you to understand the importance of protein. This is not a protein-only book. This is not the Atkins Diet that was made popular years ago. This is just the facts of how the body functions and what is required nutritionally for that to happen.

You can lose weight, actually gain muscle, and burn fat by just changing your eating. Let me explain that to you. It is not that you are going to be eating a bunch of bad tasting stuff that you are not going to have any enjoyment in. We all want to have more energy, less fat, and better health. So do it.

Please understand the purpose of this book is to inform, educate, and hopefully motivate. If you bought this book looking for the Grapefruit 45 or Cabbage Soup fad diets, then you bought the wrong book.

When my patients asks for help to lose weight, I throw it right back at them, and I say, for one week, write down everything that is going into your body – food, drinks, supplements, and medicines. That is <u>everything</u> for one week.

Ninety percent of the time they will not do it. It requires effort. Anything that you want in this world, in your life, probably requires effort -- why is weight loss any different? The facts are that you are required to do your homework here. You are required to read labels and have a little more aware-ness of what is going into your body and how it affects you.

Proteins are essential parts of organisms. Proteins can be broken down further into things like amino acids. You have heard of insulin, but have you heard of leptin? Leptin seems to be more of an important hormone than even insulin.

The body assimilates proteins most efficiently if proteins are consumed frequently during the day. Six small meals, each containing some protein, allow the body to make better use of the nutrients than if you were to eat it at two or three large meals.

Scientists have proven that 98% of the atoms in your body are replaced within one year. Every three months or so, your body produces entirely new red blood cells. Every six weeks, all the cells are replaced in your liver, and your stomach lining are replaced every five days. You are continually replacing old blood cells with new ones. Every month producing new skin cells as dead cells are shed and new cells are grown under-neath. The proteins in your muscles are continually turned over as muscle and broken down as the new tissue is made. Every cell in your body is constantly being recycled.

Author and mind-body expert, Dr. Deepak Chopra, describes the ongoing cellular renewal process like this, "it is as if you lived in a building whose bricks were systematically taken out and replaced every year. If you keep the same blueprint, it will still look like the same building. But it won't be the same in actuality. The human body also stands there, looking much the same from day to day, but through the process of respiration, digestion, illumination and so forth, is constantly and ever in exchange with the rest of the world". From a cellular standpoint, you are not the same person you were year ago. This is important for you to understand because it makes you realize that the statement, "you are what you eat", should be taken literally. You really need to think twice about what you put in your body every day.

Protein is raw building material for the human body. If your body is constantly recycling cells, the question is where do all the cells come from? The answer, of course, is from your food, specifically protein.

Protein is the actual raw construction material for body cells like bricks are for buildings. Body structures made from protein are: skin, hair, nails, bones, connective tissue, and, of course, muscle. Mix in water, and protein is the most abundance substance in your body making up about 20% of your weight. Sixty-seven percent of all protein in the body is located in the skeletal muscles.

Like fats and carbs, proteins are also composed of carbon, hydrogen, and oxygen. It is the presence of nitrogen that separates protein from other macronutrients. Only protein can bring nitrogen into the body because muscle tissue contains most of the body's protein and protein contains nitrogen. Scientists can study the effect of dietary protein on muscle growth by comparing the nitrogen balance. If the intake of nitrogen is greater than the amount excreted, than we know that proteins are being retained. Therefore, new muscle is being synthesized. This is known as a positive-action balance. If more nitrogen is excreted than consumed, you are in negative-nitrogen balance indicating that protein is being broken down and muscle is being lost.

The small components of proteins are called amino acids. Amino acids are the building blocks of protein. Proteins are formed from the joining of numerous amino acids. There are 20 amino acids that are required for growth by the human body. From these 20 amino acids, there are tens of thousands of different protein molecules that can be formed. Each protein is assembled from the bonding of different amino acids in the various configurations. For example, growth hormone contains 156 amino acids.

Amino acids are a lot like bricks. Individual bricks are building material that can be cemented together into a nearly unlimited number of structures such as a brick house, a brick wall, a brick oven, a brick chimney, etc.

Regarding amino acids, there is what is called essential and nonessential amino acids. Out of the 20 amino acids, the body can make 11 of them. These are called non-essential amino acids. The other 9 amino acids are called essential. Essential amino acids are those, which the body cannot make and you must get in your food. For game show trivia, the essential amino acids are histodine, isoleucine, leucine, valine, lysine, methionine, phenylalanine, threonine, and tryptophan.

Foods that contain a balanced combination of all the essential and non-essential amino acids, in the exact amounts required by the body for growth, are called complete proteins. In order for the body to synthesize muscle, all the essential amino acids must be available simultaneously. The liver can produce any non-essential amino acids that are in short supply.

If an essential amino acid is missing, the body must break down its own proteins to obtain it. To prevent muscle cell breakdown, dietary protein must supply all the essential amino acids. If your diet is missing any essential amino acids, protein synthesis will be inhibited. That is why consuming protein at every meal is VITAL!

Carbs have a storage depot in the body called the glycogen area. Glycogen can be stored in the muscles and liver and then drawn upon hours or even days later as needed. Proteins cannot be stored in the body. There is only a very small and transient amino acid pool in the bloodstream. To maintain the optimal environment for muscle growth and positive nitrogen balance, complete proteins must be eaten with every meal. This is why bodybuilders eat six protein meals each day. This does not mean that you will become big and bulky from adding more protein to your meals. In fact it is the opposite. You will become leaner.

Proteins are not just found in meat, eggs, and milk. There is also protein in vegetables, beans, legumes, and whole grains. The proteins in the second group I mentioned are not considered complete because they lack one or more of the essential amino acids. The complete protein sources come from animals such as eggs, milk, and meat.

In addition, supplementation to help your protein intake can be beneficial. WHEY protein powders are an excellent source to help get your required amounts of protein. Other supplementation and amino acid supplements are helpful, but do not replace whole food choices.

A list of complete proteins are as following: chicken breast, turkey breast, fish, eggs, lean red meats, tuna, milk, and whey-based protein powders.

How much protein you need depends on your size, your activity level, your occupation, etc. Bodybuilders, for example, eat 1g of protein per pound of body weight. Most exercise coaches will tell you .8g per pound of body weight. On the low scale, you should get, at least, one third of your nutrition from protein.

If you like math, and I know you do, here is a better approach. Since we are all different sizes and shapes, do this to determine your daily intake goal of protein. If you weigh 200 pounds and have 15% body fat, that is 30 pounds of fat. Subtract that and you have your lean weight of 170. Now ask yourself the following: What is my activity level?

- Sedentary - multiply pounds of lean body weight by .5
- Light activity (e.g. walking) - multiply by .6
- Moderate (30 minutes of vigorous activity 3 days per week) multiple by .7
- Active (1 hour per day 5 days per week) multiple by .8
- Very Active (10 hours of vigorous activity per week) multiple by .9
- Athlete - multiply by 1.0

This is a great formula. People that exercise actually require more nutrition and more protein. Multiply your LEAN weight by the numbers above to give you a daily goal of protein intake.

In an article written by Dr. Mercola at mercola.com, he discusses the fact that nutrition is the answer to building stronger muscles. He states resistance exercise promotes muscle building, but just how much muscle mass you gain is variable and depends on factors including your nutritional choices. This is what I discuss with my patients. People at the gym are the ones that are trying to exercise, putting a lot of effort, but are not getting the results. You want to destroy your efforts at the gym?? Then suck down a big Gatorade right when you are done. That will slow you down faster than anything. <u>Drink your water people!</u>

Researchers noted in the *Journal of Nutrition and Metabolism* the following: "nutritional interventions designed to maximally stimulate muscle protein synthesis may be useful for those individuals concerned with enhancing skeletal muscle protein assimilation". This means simply that exercise is the spark, while nutrition is the fuel for your metabolism. You can exercise until you are blue in the face, <u>but until you master what you eat, you will never reach your true fitness potential</u>. Remember that 80 to 90% of the results of your health and physique are related to the foods you eat and do not eat. Ten to 20% of your fitness and health is related to exercise.

As I said before, at the end of this book I will be giving links for products that I use and recommend. I am completely against artificial sweeteners. Splenda and NutraSweet are a no-no! I highly recommend that everybody invest in a high-quality whey protein. This is a protein shake that you can mix with water or almond milk. To get some much needed protein. In terms of building muscle and muscle tone, whey is preferred over milk for a variety of reasons. One, research has shown whey protein is superior to other milk proteins for building muscle. It appears that the amino acids found in high-quality whey protein activate certain cellular mechanisms which in turn promote muscle protein synthesis while protecting against declining testosterone levels. Additionally, milk is loaded with lactose or milk sugar. This is a combination of glucose and galactose. Even raw, organic grass-fed milk can be a problem with others who struggle with insulin resistance. The researchers stressed that high-quality leucine rich proteins, such as whey, may be particularly important for the elderly to maximize muscle protein synthesis. Leucine is part of the branched chain amino acids that serve multiple functions in your body, one of which is signaling a mechanism to increase protein synthesis and build muscle.

Most people do not eat enough protein to maintain their muscle mass which you can lose each year as you age. That is why an increase in your protein is so important. By having more muscle mass, your body will not break down as fast and you can have less reliance on medications because you will be healthier.

Note, supplementation is not always as effective as getting them from food sources. Protein shakes can supply enough of the protein to fill in the gaps that you may be lacking. In another study published in the *Journal of Medicine and Science,* in sports and during exercise, consuming 20g of whey protein 30 minutes <u>before</u> exercise, training, or weight lifting will boost your body's metabolism for as much as 24 hours after your workout. In addition, consuming 20g <u>after</u> exercise increases both fat burning and muscle building at the same time.

Most people start their day by skipping breakfast or by having a cup of coffee and a bagel. Where is the protein your body needs to repair, grow, heal, and to be healthy?

When it comes to whey protein, you want to use a whey protein concentrate, not isolate. According to Dr. Mercola, "the whey protein isolates are devoid of nutritional cofactors including alkalizing minerals, naturally occurring vitamins, and lipids which are lost in the processing. This renders them deficient and overly pacifying unlike whole protein food concentrates which do not acidify in your body due to their alkalizing minerals. Whey protein isolates over acidify". I will talk about acidity and alkaline later.

Eggs are a great source of protein and, yes, you can eat the yolk. People worry about cholesterol and eggs. I will only mention that the cholesterol scare in this country is one of the biggest myths that coincide with the billions of dollars big corporations are getting for selling cholesterol-lowering drugs. Chicken and fish are also great sources of protein. For beef, you have to be selective, and get lean cuts or even grass-fed animal beef. Also, when shopping for beef, chicken, and eggs, it is always best to buy with no steroids and no antibiotics. Many forms of nuts and beans also have a tremendous amount of protein.

Our body uses protein constantly. We are constantly utilizing it, breaking it down, and recycling what we can. Of all the amino acids that are required for optimal health, nine amino acids are essential to our diet. We must get those from outside sources. The same as Omega 3 fatty acids in fish oil, it is essential.

Most people consume about 15% of their calories with protein. That is simply not enough. I will provide an action plan and steps for you to start you on your way to the all new, healthier, leaner you.

To summarize this chapter, proteins are a requirement. You must consume a far more amount of protein than you probably are now to insure a positive nitrogen balance. This will allow the body to produce more lean tissue and further allow your body to burn fat. Do not worry about the calories. Start adding lean protein with each meal. Your body wants to burn the fat -- let it.

In the next chapter, we will discuss carbs and I will talk about fats too -- the good fats and the bad fats. You will need less bad carbs and more good fats in your diet if you want to lose weight.

It is your health and future health. Be well!

Chapter 5

Carbohydrates

If you apply any chapter from this book, this is the chapter. Why is that? The answer is because too many carbs are what is making you fat. It is not necessarily too many calories, it is not that you do not exercise, it is the refined carbs, or processed carbs, that are doing it. The effect that it has on your overall health and well-being is substantial. The three whites are NOT the three amigos: white flour, sugar, and salt are the enemies.

What are carbs and the specific types? Well, first of all, we do need carbs to survive. Again, it is the balance that we all need. Your body uses carbs to make glucose which is the fuel and energy which helps keep everything going in your body.

Your body can use glucose immediately or it can be stored by your liver and muscles and used when needed. Carb sources are things like vegetables, whole grain breads, cereals, other grains. Carb sources containing added sugar like cakes, cookies, white breads, and sugar-sweetened beverages are what you need to avoid.

The purpose of this chapter is not to get you to avoid carbs completely, because you will not anyway. When you load carbs in our diet, it is brain food; it literally is "good mood food". Understand this quote from Dr. Michael Colgan, "the price paid for severe restriction of carbohydrates is a reduction in the body's protein stores, particularly muscle protein. This causes a significant reduction in lean tissue mass". So you cannot avoid carbs. Too many or too little creates that imbalance that must be corrected. The body will not ask you to fix it, it will take what it needs to do so.

Just as Chiropractors balance the spine and frame, your internal environment must also have a balance.

Hopefully, in this chapter, you will be able to learn about the various types of carbs and which ones are best for increasing energy and losing body fat. And also that some are beneficial and some are harmful. You will learn to distinguish between processed carbs and natural carbs, fibrous carbs, starchy carbs, and simple and complex carbs.

Unlike proteins, which are used as building materials, carbs are used for energy. Carbs are described as premium fuel, especially when exercising. Fats are also used for fuel. The difference is that fats do not burn as carbs do. Fat is stored in the body as a backup energy source. It is your body's reserve fuel tank. For example, a 185-pound man with 18% body fat has over 1,000 calories stored in his reserve tank. Your body can store carbs, but in much more limited quantities.

Your body is always burning a mixture of carbs and fat for fuel during low intensity, long-duration exercise. Your body can easily use mostly fat for fuel and, even in lean people, there is enough fat stored to last a long time.

The right quantity of carbs is equally important as to the quality. A carb is not a carb, they are not all the same. Do not assume that if you were to consume 500 calories of broccoli or 500 calories of soda, that the effect on the body is the same. This is why calories in and calories out is ineffective for long term weight management and loss.

There are simple and complex carbs, also starchy carbs, processed carbs, high glycemic, low glycemic index carbs, etc. The good carbs, which should be your best friends, are like real best friends. They are always there for you and reliable. They will give you energy and help you to get leaner and muscular. The bad carbs are your enemies. They are like the crazy cousin that you feel you should see and hangout with once in a while, but afterwards you feel like that was a mistake. You are dragged down and think, I will not be doing that again. These carbs have a greater potential for fat storage, they are nutritionally void, and rob you of all of your energy, among other things.

To lose fat, become leaner, regulate your metabolism, and increase your energy, understanding the different types of carbs, and their effects, will maximize your efforts.

Simple carbs consist of a single sugar molecule or two single sugar molecules together. The simple sugar is known as a monosaccharide, and the two singles together are a disaccharide. These include fructose, glucose, and galactose.

Fructose is the type found in fruit. Most fruits are ok if you eat the fruits with the skins. Fruit juice alone is not ok. Consuming milk, orange juice, or other juice will increase your chances of being overweight. Eating organic fruit, with the skin whenever possible, will neutralize the sugar content and not create an insulin response.

Lactose, which is really milk sugar, is a combination of galactose and glucose. Most simple sugars, due to their simple structure, are digested very quickly and they cause a rapid rise in blood sugar. Your body responds to the blood sugar by releasing large muscle insulin, which I will talk about in a minute.

When there is a large blood sugar spike, your body tends to overreact and produce too much insulin. The insulin quickly clears the glucose from the bloodstream leading to a sharp drop in blood sugar known as hypoglycemia. Blood sugar drops are accompanied by cravings, hunger, weakness, mood swings, and decreased energy. The hunger and cravings tend to cause the sugar consumption to perpetuate itself, resulting in a vicious cycle of ups and downs throughout the day.

For example, if you decide to skip breakfast, grab a cup of coffee and head to work. Typically then by 9 or 10 o'clock you are looking for a doughnut or a bagel. Then you feel good until lunchtime, at which time your blood sugar crashes, and you are out looking again for a quick fix that is typically fast food.

To lose body fat and burn fat more efficiently, your goal is to maintain steady blood sugar levels and here is why. The over secretion of insulin activates fat storage in cells and promotes the movement of triglycerides in the bloodstream into fat cells for storage. High insulin levels also inhibit enzymes that mobilize the breakdown of existing stored body fat. You can manage your blood sugar levels by choosing fewer simple carbs, more complex carbs, and by eating your good carbs with lean protein approximately every three hours.

Insulin is honestly not the bad guy all the time, but it is a fat storage hormone. Insulin is an anabolic hormone that is essential for getting amino acids in the muscles for growth. Anabolic means a growth or synthesis. Catabolic is the opposite, or a breakdown of tissues. The problem occurs when there is too much insulin. When resistance to insulin is produced by eating too many simple and processed carbs, and when your blood sugar insulin levels are normally high, you are not in a fat-burning mode, you are in fat-storage mode.

Insulin is a promoter of fat synthesis. But it is also a crucial hormone for promoting protein synthesis, reducing protein degradation (including suppressing cortisol, which can be catabolic in nature), and promoting glucose uptake and glycogen storage in muscle. Insulin, notably, also suppresses appetite.

The bottom line is that you must control your blood sugar or it will control you. When you get to my Action Plan portion of this book, you will be consuming nutrition where you will not have to count calories, but rather it is designed to regulate and normalize your blood sugar and insulin sensitivity.

When I talk about simple carbs, I am referring to the refined and processed white flour products. These are the bad carbs. Some of the simple carbs that occur in nature are not all bad. Fructose as those found in fruit. These are ok typically when consumed as a fruit, and not just in fruit juice. The fruit's skin, or fiber, acts as a neutralizing agent for a blood sugar spike that can occur with fruit juices alone. I will discuss juicing later, and why juicing daily, or frequently, is a nice compliment to your healthier lifestyle. You cannot simply juice fruits without affecting your blood sugar.

You need to cut out all of your simple carbs. At the very least, you should drastically reduce your simple carbs if you want maximum fat loss. This is one of the tricks body builders use to get lean. They remove refined sugar completely, even cut back on natural sugars, and replace them with starchy and fibrous carbs instead.

When fat loss is your goal, and you are watching your type of calories closely, drinking a large portion of carbs is not a good idea. Whole foods have more fiber, a low calorie density, and a higher thermic effect. Thermic effect means the effort and energy your body needs to digest food. It is important to eat more of your calories than drink them, as this revs the metabolism.

The other side of simple carbs is what is called complex carbs. Complex carbs are broken down into starchy and fibrous categories. These carbs take longer to breakdown and digest which has a higher thermic effect. Starchy carbs are found in potatoes, cereals, grains, bread, pasta, rice, oats, wheat, and beans.

Fiber is the indigestible portion of food or plants that passes straight through your digestive tract without all the energy being absorbed. Fiber promotes healthy digestion, elimination, speeds the transit time of food to the intestinal tract, and provides protection from gastrointestinal diseases and colon cancer. You could say that fiber is nature's internal cleanser – it is very important. I recommend Psyllium seeds to be mixed in with your protein shakes.

Fibrous carbs, such as green vegetables are your BFFs (best friends forever). They have a low-calorie density. Low-calorie dense foods are great for fat loss because they make it easier to stay full. It is very possible, from consuming a ton of green veggies, which you will get tired of chewing before you eat too much.

Complex carbs should make up the majority of your carb calories, because they take longer to digest and absorb than the simple carbs. They contain fiber, which slows down the absorption, and help stabilize blood sugar and insulin. Whereas refined, or processed carbs, are nutritionally void, spike blood sugar, and tell your body to store fat.

Understand that a processed carb converts in the body just as sugar does. They are equal. Here are 12 reasons to avoid processed foods and sugar.
1. Refined sugar can be a contributing factor to gain body fat.
2. Increases the bad cholesterol.
3. Decreases the good cholesterol.
4. Increases triglycerides and fats.

5. Suppresses your immune system. (As a Chiropractor when patients tell me them or a family member are sick, I tell them to avoid sugar. <u>Sugar feeds the bug</u>. It is like a stray cat, if you leave food for it, it will keep coming back.)
6. Depletes your body of important minerals.
7. Contributes to the development of cancers.
8. Causes hypoglycemia. (This is low blood sugar and a pre-cursor to diabetes.)
9. Decreases growth hormone. (The biggest mistake after a workout is grabbing a sugary drink. You might as well not have worked out. Your post work-out meal is an extension of your workout. Stick with water or a whey protein shake immediately after a workout for better results.)
10. Contributes to diabetes and heart disease.
11. May cause food allergies. (Another side note, you should also cycle your proteins and foods around. This helps with boredom, but also helps with food allergies and will help assimilate and process foods better.)
12. Increases insulin secretions. (more pre-diabetes and fat storage.)

Sure I can list more, but the threat of fat storage, diabetes, heart disease, and cancers should be enough to make you avoid the drive thru for a while.

Your carb consumption based on grams, should be a total of 50% of your daily calorie intake. This is baseline and subject to tweaking. Exercise levels and activity levels may require greater consumption. Also keep in mind, that these recommendations are for fat loss, not weight maintenance, weight gain or, athletic performance.

The healthier foods include ones that provide dietary fiber, with some whole grains, as well as those without sugars. The distinctive foods like sodas and candies that have added sugars, means extra calories, but not many nutrients. Specifically, <u>you should avoid anything that has high fructose corn syrup added.</u>

I am sure by now that you understand there is a difference between good carbs and bad carbs. The best way to shop at the grocery store is to stay on the outer of the store.

The isles in the middle are the man-made stuff and should be off limits.

You may also see when you are looking at food labels that fiber is either soluble or insoluble. Soluble is found in oatmeal, most fruits, beans and peas. Insoluble fiber will be found in whole-wheat bread, brown rice, wheat bran, most vegetables, and some fruits.

Soluble fibers attract water and form a gel, which slows down digestion. Soluble fiber delays the emptying of your stomach and makes you feel full, which helps control weight. Slower stomach emptying may also affect blood sugar levels and have a beneficial effect on insulin sensitivity, which may help control diabetes. Soluble fibers can also help lower LDL ("bad") blood cholesterol by interfering with the absorption of dietary cholesterol.

Insoluble fibers are considered gut-healthy fiber because they have a laxative effect and add bulk to the diet, helping prevent constipation. These fibers do not dissolve in water, so they pass through the gastrointestinal tract relatively intact, and speed up the passage of food and waste through your gut. Insoluble fibers are mainly found in whole grains and vegetables.

Most Americans do not have a sufficient amount of dietary fiber. Breads, rolls, or pizza made with refined flour are not the best sources of dietary fiber. They, unfortunately, contribute to a large portion of the American diet. It is recommended that you get about 14g of dietary fiber for every 1,000 calories consumed each day.

Here are some tips if you want get some adequate fiber in your diet. Choose whole fruits versus fruit juice. Try to eat vegetables with your evening meal. Keep a bowl of vegetables in your refrigerator, things like carrots, cucumbers, or celery for a quick snack. Make one meal around dried beans, peas, or legumes instead of meat.

That is why it is important to recognize things such as the glycemic index and glycemic load. It not only is about how fast something converts in the body, but the effect it has on us.

The glycemic index is a measure of how quickly food glucose is absorbed and will raise your blood sugar. The glycemic load estimates the impact of carb consumption using the glycemic index, while taking into account the amount of carbs that are consumed. For instance, watermelon has a high glycemic index, but a typical serving of watermelon does not contain much carbs, so the glycemic effect of eating it (and, therefore, its glycemic load) is low.

The simple carbs, or processed carbs, are the most addicting substances that you can put in your body. When we think of addictions, we think of alcohol and drugs. Sugar is actually one of the most addicting substances. It has an addiction cycle and process. Your brain has what is called the pleasure-reward system. How it essentially works is when you put sugar in your body and it tastes incredibly good, your brain will seek more. If you are reading this book and overweight, than you have been giving your body too much sugar and need to start fueling the body versus feeding the body.

There is a story about an experiment regarding a frog in a pot of water. If you were to take a pot of water and bring it to boil, and drop a frog in the pot of water, it will be so hot that the frog will jump out. This is a protective mechanism by the frog. If you took the same frog, placed it in water that was at room temperature, and turned on the stove so that the temperature would slowly rise, the frog would not detect the small increases in temperature, and would be cooked alive. Whether this story is an actual experiment or just a tale, it makes a great point. You see yourself every day. You do not detect the small changes that occur within your body. I have seen patients in my office after not seeing them for six months and they put on 20 pounds during that time. Many go from a youthful appearance, to old looking in a very short time.

I have been saying this to my patients for years, "don't be the frog!" Remember, "it's not what you do all the time, it's what you do most of the time that matters". Health is cumulative. If you choose to burn the candle at both ends, it will catch up with you.

This is your life we are talking about. <u>There are no do-overs</u>. If you chronically live on sodas, breads, and junk food you will pay for it. If you join a large corporate weight loss company, where it is a point system and you starve yourself all day, then have a Big Mac, fries and a Coke, you are good, right? As long as the "points" are good, then I can eat that, right? – WRONG!!! The body does not work that way.

You can still have fun food sometimes, if you follow the rule that you are good MOST OF THE TIME. I am giving you the basics. I am laying down a foundation. This book is the basics. We all need to get back to the basics. I will spell out a plan for you to get on track, or get you back on track.

To use an example, let us look at college basketball legend, Coach Bobby Knight. Everyone remembers Bobby Knight for throwing a chair across the floor. What most do not recognize is that he is one of the greatest coaches ever. He almost never had incredible players. But what he understood is the basics of the game. He broke the game down to the basic levels, like taking high percentage shots and making more free throws than the other team attempted.

Let me compare that with Chiropractic. Chiropractic is so simple in its understanding that people have a hard time believing that it can work. Your spine protects the spinal nerves, and when the spine is misaligned, it affects nerve and blood flow which results in symptoms. Restore the motion, remove nerve pressure, and the body can heal. It is so simple. However for weight loss, people want the short cuts, people prefer to medicate, inject, or elect for surgery. Short cuts rarely work.

If you are serious about losing weight and getting thinner, then you are going to have to limit your bad carb intake greatly. Sodas and sugary drinks are out. Diet drinks, milk, and juices are out. Some of you are right now thinking I cannot do that. Yes you can! You do not think you can because it is a habit for you and your body is addicted to sugar. Most people in this country burn sugar, but never burn fat.

When you eat a piece of bread, your body looks at it as pure sugar. Your body breaks down the sugar and transports it into your bloodstream. The amount of sugar (glucose) that is in your bloodstream is toxic and it needs to get out and get into your cells. Your pancreas releases insulin to help remove the blood sugar from the bloodstream and transport it to the cells for energy. As you continue this cycle of too many carbs, your body will not respond as well and, therefore, you have insulin sensitivity. Meaning that either there is not enough insulin to go around because of your increased weight, or the majority of insulin is not as effective in moving the glucose from the blood.

Diabetes is a very real problem. Adult-onset diabetes, or Type II, is what I am discussing, which is the majority of diabetes cases in this country. That is the one that is <u>not</u> insulin dependent. Type I requires injections of insulin, and is a pancreas issue. <u>Type II is nutritionally reversible. Let me say that again, Type II is nutritionally reversible!</u>

If being overweight, feeling tired, and having joint pain is not enough, what about the very real possibility of losing a foot or having a leg removed below the knee?

The importance of controlling insulin production cannot be understated. It is the hormone responsible for fat storage and is the only one over which we have complete control. It is important to think twice before deviating, even slightly, from a well-designed nutritional plan. The reasons for this become clearer when you consider some of the ways in which insulin inhibits fat loss.

Insulin is a storage hormone, not only the storage of sugar, but also that of fats and magnesium. Elevated insulin levels prompt increased fat storage, but will also increase feelings of low energy by reducing the amount of magnesium in circulation. Magnesium supports production of what is called ATP. ATP is the body's energy molecule. It also increases the production of what is called lipoprotein lipase, which is an enzyme to break down fat, or triglycerides, in the blood stream for storage.

Insulin also inhibits what is called carnitine. Carnitine is needed to escort fat from the fat cells to the mitochondria. Mitochondria are these little cellular organs that are located in every cell. They produce ATP, which is our energy in a process called the Krebs cycle.

I hated biochemistry, but the bottom line is that high insulin prevents fat from being used as an energy source. So again, it is not that you just had a cookie, cake, or soda with too many calories, it is the effect of the blood sugar and insulin response from them.

I have friends that will exercise before a night of beer drinking. Or think it is ok to have a bunch of pizza, because they are jogging five miles tomorrow. The fact is, is not ok.

You know that bloated feeling? High insulin tells the kidneys to hold onto the sodium causing the retention of water. This increased retention adds a bloated appearance, which also raises your blood pressure to increase blood volume.

Blood pressure is also raised by insulin's affect on each adrenal glands. The adrenal glands are stress glands. What happens when you are eating so much garbage, you gain weight, and your blood pressure goes up? The first medication that your medical doctor will prescribe for you is a diuretic to release fluids within the body to lower the pressure.

The importance of controlling your blood sugar, and its associated effect on insulin production, can be easily seen as a main purpose of this book. We want your body to become in balance. <u>Remember, the nutritional component is completely controlled by you by making the right food choices, the more you do that, the more rapidly you will increase the level of your success.</u>

Look, no one should become obsessed with labels and counting calories. You should familiarize yourself with what you are eating. Highly processed foods are out. You do not need to go cold turkey, but more power if you can.

The first thing you do start with portion control. If every Friday night you come home with a large pizza, then next Friday get a small one. If you are sucking down a 2-liter of soda every week, cut that in half the next week.

Eventually I want you to set goals, and tell yourself by the end of this month, or within 30 days, I am going to have no more soda. I am going to have pizza once a month as a reward.

You can do it. It may not be easy all the time. Sometimes it is going to be incredibly easy. You are going to shock even yourself. Remember, food is like a drug. You may experience withdrawal symptoms, especially if you drink a lot of caffeine and suddenly decrease that amount or eliminate it altogether. A cool T-shirt I saw said, "Pain is just weakness leaving the body".

So, when you are going through this process of transforming over the next several months, think of a headache or fatigue as your body's way of getting rid of toxins and setting yourself up for a new, healthier you.

When I talk about a chapter of carbs, what I am really meaning is the effect of carbs and what the body does in response.

I will caution you that a lot of people have switched from white bread to whole-wheat bread. I would say that a grain is still a grain for the most part. Whole-wheat bread may not have the blood sugar response as quickly as white bread, but it still has a response and it is still a grain. Personally, I would avoid grains altogether. With genetically modified crops and gluten sensitivity adding to our waistlines and health problems, avoiding them altogether seems appropriate.

When you start to implement my advice, spend at least two to three weeks with no grains of any kind. This will allow your insulin sensitivity to regulate faster and also reduce your sugar cravings.

Sometimes we try to make healthier choices, but it is just the appearance of healthier choices. For example, drinking diet soda versus regular soda, in many ways diet soda is worse for you. They both have similar chemicals. Regular has high fructose corn syrup and diet has artificial sweeteners, like Splenda and NutraSweet, which are neurotoxins (cancer causing) and should be avoided. Just drink water!

People go to the store and buy things that are fat-free or sugar-free. Yet as a country, we are heavier than we were 20 years ago, even 10 years ago. I wish we had a different name for fats. We could just call people overweight versus fat because fats have a bad rap.

In the next chapter I will discuss fats and the importance of good fats in our diet. <u>Again fats do not make us fat, carbs do.</u>

If you find yourself having difficulty losing weight after modifying your diet, then checking your insulin and leptin levels would be beneficial. It is really all about regulating your internal environment to function exactly how it was designed. The body can naturally produce painkillers, muscle relaxers, and ant-inflammatories if you fuel it correctly.

To summarize this chapter, the avoidance of simple carbs will help control and regulate your insulin and leptin productions so your body does not store excess calories as fat, but rather burns fat as fuel. The longer you negatively affect your blood sugar levels to go up and down, the greater the chance you have for obesity, heart disease, diabetes, and cancers.

You must understand that I am talking about YOUR health. It is yours – not mine. This starts with YOU. If you are eating poorly and gaining weight, and you have young children, then they are probably eating like this as well. Nobody wants their kids to be overweight and unhealthy. Make the choices yourself and give it time. You probably have been eating like this for years, please give it some time to regulate.

You can still have a beer, slice of pizza, or a glass of wine occasionally. Make it a conscious choice when you want something and call it a reward, just do not do it every day. Never have back-to-back meals that are poor. Again, "it's not what you do all of the time, it's what you do most of the time that matters".

Be healthy for today and tomorrow.

Chapter 6

Insulin

In the last chapter I discussed carbs, probably to exhaustion. Sorry, I know it was long, but it was all really important information. Now, you cannot discuss carbs without discussing insulin, which I did somewhat in the last chapter. But here goes insulin's own chapter.

When you understand the facts of how you have such great control over your health and weight loss, you will start to make better choices. I have said it before, and you know I will say it again -- "it's not what you do all the time, it's what you do most the time that matters".

Please do not take that statement and try to play around with it. Like, wow I have eaten good two meals today, so now I can pig out on my third meal. No! What that means is, if you take care yourself and you do some things that I am teaching you in this book, you can still enjoy your favorite foods. If you want to lose weight, and have a lean figure, you have to make changes and sacrifices.

Let me give an example. My good friends have kids. They keep mentioning that they really need to sign one of them up for some sport because she is getting fat. They have repeated this statement many times. Their daughter is 11 years old and lives on soda. Of course soda is loaded with sugar and caffeine. They also comment on her being hyper all the time – gee, I wonder why? Sadly, it is not the lack of activity making her fat; it is the soda that is doing it. Her health is getting destroyed from soda. No one should drink soda, certainly not a child with a growing, developing body. But, it is all an insulin-related response that is controllable.

Insulin is a hormone produced in the pancreas. It is a storage hormone. When you eat your food, your body breaks it down and the nutrients, or lack thereof, enter the bloodstream. The converted food to be used as fuel must be taken out of the bloodstream and get used by the cells. Insulin is what is released for this to occur.

Insulin is secreted when blood glucose rises after eating a meal. Insulin assists in regulating blood sugar by transporting the glucose into muscle, cells, and other tissues, as well as to the liver. Glucose fuels the muscles, red blood cells, and fat tissues. It is stored in the liver as glycogen for future use. Blood sugar transported to fat tissues is stored as fat. When insulin is secreted, the cells absorb the glucose from the blood. The high blood glucose is then lowered to a normal range. Glucagon is the hormone that is the opposite of insulin. Pancreatic cells also secrete it. If the blood glucose is high, glucagon is not secreted. However, when blood glucose is low, for example between meals or even while exercising, glucagon is secreted.

You may have tried to exercise for five days week to lose weight and have had limited, to no success. Many people want to lose that last 5 or 10 pounds. Those people still have no luck. Have you ever wondered why? The answer is insulin sensitivity.

Insulin sensitivity is also synonymous with weight loss or fat loss. Insulin has a powerful ability to prevent fat breakdown because of its anabolic or rebuilding properties. Anabolic is like an anabolic steroid, creating big muscles. Anabolic means building. The opposite is catabolic which is a break down.

Most doctors, professionals, and even fitness experts have no clue about insulin sensitivity and the effects it has on our desire for fat loss. I have a membership to a chain of gyms throughout the country that has cardio equipment, weight machines, tanning beds, etc. All the locations I have been to all seem to have a trainer within the gym. The problem with most of these trainers is that they are teaching old school techniques and they offer zero, none, zilch in terms of nutritional advice or modifications. Listen to me when I tell you, <u>you will never have any sustained weight loss without nutritional modifications</u>. I do not want to hear people say, "Oh I can eat whatever I want as long as I go to the gym, I will just burn it off". Sorry folks, it does not work that way. I do not want you to simply lose weight; I want you to truly become healthier.

You probably know somebody who never works out, eats whatever they want, and has a perfect physique. Well guess what, there are exceptions to the rule, and, frankly, there are a few lucky people out there that won the genetic lottery.

So I will explain insulin's role again, and how its changes will affect your weight and essentially fat loss. What most people do not realize is that insulin targets the fat cells when it is released. Research tells us that insulin sensitivity is actually increased when you lower your weight or your body fat percentage. Also that insulin sensitivity gets stronger the more you workout. The catabolic effect of exercise increases insulin sensitivity during a workout and for about 30 to 45 minutes after your workout. This means as a healthy, exercising individual, you must constantly tweak and modify your nutrition.

You have all heard the definition of "insanity" correct? It is doing the same thing over and over again, but expecting different results. Look, I have been there. I promise you and guarantee that nobody will out discipline me, ever. I was – was the guy at the gym who could spend hours on the treadmill, elliptical or stationary bike. I would leave a big pool of my sweat too. Oh, and if you came next to me, I would stay there until you left. I had to prove a point. The point is, I was not helping my body in the long run. Slow cardio and long distances is actually catabolic. I ran five marathons, so I know what it does to the body.

What I never had was that lean muscular physique. I could go to the gym every day, but I never got lean and fit until I understood the role of nutrition, insulin sensitivity, and its affect on how the body stores and burns fat. Today is much different.

It is important to note that insulin is sensitive to both carbs and protein consumed, not fat consumed. However, of all the food sources, it is the carb meals that elevate insulin levels the most. If you really want to raise your insulin levels, stick with high fructose corn syrup as a staple in your diet and I guarantee you will have major health problems. Just like my friend's daughter and soda.

I will talk about high fructose corn syrup in a minute. But, if you want a top 10 list of how your body and health is going to be affected by high fructose corn syrup, here it is: obesity, diabetes, tooth decay, bad cholesterol, tri-glycerides increase, increase risk of heart attack and heart disease, anemia, lowered immunity, lack of good calories, fatigue, mood swings, and depression.

I mentioned above that insulin sensitivity is increased when healthier. Why would your body become more sensitive as you become healthier? It is very simple – survival. Your body is an adaptive machine. It adapts or it dies. Just like an animal has a thicker coat of fur in the winter, your body will actually store more fat during the cold weather – that is survival.

Try to imagine this; the body has a way to protect itself. I want to repeat this example, as many of my patients still do not believe me. Maybe you do not as well. Let us use this example of the calories in/calories out model of weight loss. We know that 3500 calories burned equals one-pound loss. There are 52 weeks in a year, and let us say the first 2 weeks of the year, we do not burn nor gain any calories. During the remaining 50 weeks, we burn an extra 3500 cal per week. In this example a person had a starting weight of 200 pounds. Burning one pound per week for 50 weeks equals 50 pounds. Therefore, at the end of one year they should weigh 150 pounds. Take that model and apply it to the second year, so now they are going to weigh 100 pounds? Let us go again for the third year. Are you thinking that this person is only going to weigh 50 pounds?

From an article written in Health.com by Cynthia Sass called Six Diet Myths Busted. I am quoting a few paragraphs: "Researchers found that when calories were limited, levels of cortisol, a stress hormone, rose. Calorie counting, even without limitations, also made the women more stressed. Cortisol is known to rev up appetite, spike cravings for fatty and sugary foods, and lead to an increase in belly fat, so causing it to surge surely isn't a smart weight-control strategy.

There are three types of calories your body needs: carbs, protein, and fat. Because each performs a unique function, they aren't interchangeable, so getting the right amount of each is important. For example, if you ate too few protein calories and too many carb calories, the jobs that proteins do wouldn't get done, and the surplus carb calories would get sent straight to your fat cells.

This can result in weight gain, as well as the loss of muscle mass, dry, dull hair and skin, hormonal imbalances, and a weaker immune system. Too much or too little of all three calorie types can lead to unwanted side effects. So getting a certain number of daily calories, without regard to the type of food, just doesn't make sense.

For these reasons and the others above, I've seen clients start to eat more calories and finally break a weight loss plateau and achieve real and lasting results. I'm not saying to ignore calories completely, but don't obsess over them. Instead, choose more fresh foods or foods as close to their natural state as possible. Strive for a balance of "good" carbs, lean protein and healthy fats to help your body function optimally. Eat breakfast every day to jump-start your metabolism, eat on a regular schedule, spacing your meals about 3-5 hours apart. Pay attention as you eat and stop when you feel just full enough, satisfied, energized and ready to move on with your day. When you listen, your body is pretty good at telling you how much it needs, no math required."

So to get back to what I was saying before. If a body has a 500-calorie deficit, it would just keep losing weight, without any self-correcting system, and would then be in danger of wasting itself away.

The human body is much smarter than you are. It will slow down its own metabolism; it will use bone, muscle, and other tissues as a food source if you restrict its consumption.

As I am writing this chapter, I had a report with a patient today. A 27 year-old man trying to get in shape, dedicated 100%, works out one hour each day with weights and circuit training, and takes all the popular supplements. He informed me that he consumes about 800 calories per day. Does anyone think that this is enough? He wonders why he cannot lose weight and burn the fat. He needs to read my book.

Of course, you could try a fad and drastically reduce your calories, or go ahead and get injected with HCG and have that be your solution for weight loss. HCG stands for human chorionic gonadatrphin. It is the hormone that is produced by a pregnant woman. It is the reason why the home pregnancy kits turn the stick blue, or positive, when pregnant. When you drastically reduce calories as I have mentioned, your body will look for a food source. The theory (myth) with HCG, is that with these injections, it will trick your body into not using muscle tissue and bone and, therefore, you can essentially starve yourself and lose weight without becoming a yo-yo dieters. This is false and unsafe. Do not do that.

Sometimes when you are desperate, you make rash decisions. If you do not stand for something, you will fall for anything. Sadly, many M.D.'s and D.C.'s offer HCG drops or injections. The only benefit it has is to the person selling it.

You understand that people who do these fads, or yo-yo dieting, eventually hurt their body in the long run, and that is why they gain more weight back from when they started. If you have fallen for the HCG gimmick, I feel bad for you because you have wasted your money. I have seen patients try HCG and starve themselves. They end up putting the weight back on and now have more loose skin. It is very similar to a gastric bypass-type surgery. I will talk about all these things later and why you should try a healthier approach.

So to get back to what I was saying before. If a body has a 500 calorie deficit, it would just keep losing weight, without any self-correcting system, and would then be in danger of wasting itself away.

If your body were not able to adjust, soft tissues, such as ligaments, tendons, and muscles, would be uncontrolled and weak. The shutting down of vital systems in the body is what would happen next.

There is plenty of evidence that restriction of calories does not allow the body to recycle and repair. We see osteoporosis, degrees of vision problems, and bone and joint problems. The evidence is out there and suggests the body leeches, or takes nutrients, from other parts of itself, if it is not obtained from the diet. Without a rebuilding response from the body, it would be unable to get bigger and stronger or recover properly from exercise stress.

Insulin's role is a protective role to maintain the integrity of internal systems as well as keeping energy stores at an optimal and safe level. Insulin is a very good protective system. But like all systems, it can be manipulated. Insulin sensitivity is a pre-program mechanism responded to the amount of sweetness in the carbs that we eat.

Everybody has a unique set of levels, which are governed by many internal factors that can be measured by determining your metabolic type. Some people have a lower insulin sensitivity level, while some have a higher insulin sensitivity level. If your body has a slow responding insulin response, you can eat more carbs without gaining weight and having negative effects. If you have a high level of insulin response, then you need to retrain it to go the other way, because almost looking at a carb will make you fat.

This is why at the end of my book I am going to give you a nutritional program for the first few weeks. What I am going to do is reboot your system. Just like if your computer freezes and you need to restart it. I am going to help restart your insulin sensitivity.

What this chapter comes down to is that our bodies have become stubborn fat burners. Our bodies are still capable of burning fat, but you need to restart your system and flip that switch. For most of us, our bodies have learned to primarily burn sugar and store fat. Guess what, you do not need that many carbs to survive. Cakes, cookies, bread, bagels, and pizza all taste wonderful, but just do not eat them every day.

The brain is really the only part of your body needs carbs. But again, it does not need the carbs I listed above. The rest your body is really happy using fat as energy. Clearly our bodies are built to run on fat and use carbs sparingly; otherwise our anatomy would be completely different. It would be like building a car with a tiny fuel tank. It would make more sense to design a car with a much bigger fuel tank with a richer fuel supply.

We consume too much sugar in this country. We stick our kids out on the baseball field where he stands in right field for 20 minutes and does not move, then goes in to sit on the bench for 20 minutes, before he could swing at three balls and sit down or maybe run or walk to first. What does he get after the game? Gatorade - sugar water. Fruit juice drinks and flavored water is nothing but sugar too. <u>Just give them water!</u>

And please do not tell me that you are a smarter parent because you use things like Splenda and NutraSweet. Those two are artificial sweeteners. I will tell you that if you use Splenda or NutraSweet, or any other artificial sweeteners, you are unhealthy. Artificial sweeteners are classified as neurotoxins. They negatively affect your nervous system and negatively affect blood sugar. They will actually make you heavier versus thinner. There are numerous studies that link artificial sweetener toxicity with a host of symptoms from migraine headaches, irritable bowel syndrome, high blood pressure, <u>and many cancers</u>.

The further we get away from nature, the more likely you are going to be a typical, overweight, unhealthy American -- osteoporotic, with diabetes, heart disease, joint pain, and cancer. I said it before and I will say it again, this is your health, not mine, it is yours. I have seen way too many people treat their dogs better than they treat their own kids and themselves. Example of friends of ours, they feed their dogs on a regular schedule. The same amount of organic food for their pets and no table scraps. Yet their kids have grown up on soda, Gatorade, box cereals, and fast food. They seem to wonder why their kids are sick all time (and of course mine are not).

I see people in the gym all the time that train, train, train, and train, but yet their body never changes. For the most part, and I will talk about this at the end of the book, but when people do make the effort to exercise, they do not do it correctly. For the most part, they do not exercise hard enough. Then, after three or four weeks of no changes in their physique, they quit. <u>It all comes down to nutrition</u>.

In comparison, there are other people that I know who eat clean. Raw vegetables, they cook most of their meals at home, and avoid heavily processed foods. Remember, it is much easier to over indulge with too many calories in your food, than it is to work it off at the gym.

Briefly, to over emphasize, if you do not provide your body with adequate nutritional support, you will start experiencing sicknesses, lethargy, and fatigue. Continue to ignore this and you get joint problems and bone problems. In fact, back to the diet drinks (with artificial sweeteners), we call diet drinks "osteoporosis in a can". Sodas, and especially diet sodas, contain an ingredient called phosphoric acid. Because it is so acidic, the body has to neutralize the acidity and bring you back to more of an alkaline or neutral state. The way this occurs is the body takes calcium from your bones to neutralize the effects of the phosphoric acid and, therefore, you make weaker bones. I guarantee your medical doctor does not know that, nor do they care.

The leaching of nutrients from your other body parts or other systems, to compensate for your lack of nutrition, malnutrition, or toxicity, will only serve to weaken you as a whole. This makes it harder and harder to function and keep in a healthy state were all your systems are working synergistically to burn fat.

Please understand that the human body is the greatest machine ever invented. What happens to this incredible machine is that WE get in its way. Most people are just too toxic. That is why there has been a big push to sell water systems that not only clean and purify your water, but the water is considered alkaline. Alkaline-based water systems can move the body from toxicity to more of a neutral state. You cannot just drink alkaline-based water.

As a Chiropractor, I have been solicited to sell things like Xangosteen, Mangosteen, Xri, Goji Berries, and too many others that I do not remember them all. These are multi-level marketing companies, where the only people that make money, are the people at the top. People have claimed such outrageous health benefits. Now, I am sure that they offer some sort of benefit, but it is the "just pop a pill" mentality. It is like a flu shot. Do not take any responsibility for your health, and just got get a "magic" shot.

If the body is without certain nutrients, it takes what it needs from another part of the body. This means a further breakdown when you are already in a catabolic state. This puts a lot of stress on an already stressed body. This, of course, can release another hormone, cortisol, the stress hormone. So what are some of the fancy companies and marketers trying to do? Well, they will sell you a pill to counteract the effects of cortisol, so again it is a "magic" pill to help you chase symptoms away or chase a complex problem way. The body is more complex than that and requires more than just popping a pill or supplement to make your body more efficient.

So how do you know if your body's insulin is sensitive or not. Well, you can pretty much guarantee that your body is not functioning well if you are overweight. If you find yourself skipping breakfast and arriving at work craving a bagel or doughnut, and then a few hours later you need another sugary beverage or food while having mood swings, or find yourself sluggish, then you are probably insulin sensitive.

Just assume that you are. If you are not thin and lean, you have probably mismanaged your body and nutritional intake for a long time. Guess what? You can fix it! You can reverse it! It is all up to you! You do not have to be the person that eats fast food five days a week, and suddenly goes to nothing but raw vegetables. You need to make changes, small steps, or one large step, to improve your health.

I still eat pizza and I plan on it. However, I do not do it every day. I have my insulin and blood sugar under control. My nutrition has afforded me leanness and a lower percentage of body fat. If you handle your nutrition, then your nutrition will handle you.

The most important thing to do is a food journal. For one week write down everything that you put in your body: food, beverages, and even medications. Give yourself an honest look at what you are consuming. Just a food journal alone may be enough to open your eyes to say, I had no idea I was eating that much.

When you do a food journal, put a column next to the food and see how you felt that day, the next day, and so on. Oh sure everybody likes comfort food, but you need to see how it affects you. How it affects your mood, how it affects your sleep, performance at work, etc.

The next time you want to run out for lunch and have that burger, shake and fries remember this, you will create a very fast insulin response that tells your body I want you store most of this as fat. Since drive-thru food is devoid of nutrients, you are telling your body to go ahead and take some liver cells, muscle cells and bone cells, and use that for food. I want to be able to get to the point in my life where I bend over one day and fracture my hip (a little exaggerated), but I think you get the point.

It is sad that as we get older, it seems most of you are about running to doctors to get examined for this, a test for that, a pill here and pill there. You really do not have to go through all that. Certainly injuries, accidents, serious health issues require medical care intervention. The main point is, that if we take care of ourselves and understand that 95% of what happens to our health is nutritionally based, we can live with quality and quantity.

Write this down and look at it often. "Nothing tastes as good as thin and fit feels".

To summarize this chapter control your insulin or it will control you. Be very aware of what your food choices do to your body. Understand that you can break the cycle and restart and reboot your system. You must give it time.

It is your health. It is your future. Be there healthy.

Chapter 7

Fads

In the last few chapters I discussed on a basic level carbs, proteins, and insulin. In this chapter I am going away from that, and I want to discuss fads. Understand that this book is not a diet. You cannot spell the word "diet", without the word "die". I want you to truly become healthier. I want you to lose weight, but not at the expense of your future health.

I have a friend that has a terrible, high-stress job that he hates. When he is not working, he winds down with comfort food. As a result he is obese. I completely understand that, I have been there too. That is a main reason I wrote this book. He says he does not go to the gym anymore because he is so tired after work and stressed out. So, when he gets home, it is beer and junk food. The problem is that he skips breakfast, eats crap all day, and then wonders why his energy sucks. He has created this cycle. He must break it or it will break him.

Very clearly, please understand what I am about to tell you. You must eat to survive. You do not have to starve yourself and diet to lose weight. I am shocked at what people do to themselves to lose weight. If you truly want to lose weight you will!

There are large corporate weight loss companies that you can join, like: Jenny Craig, NutriSystem, and many others. It amazes me how similar their commercials are. It is either the really awful black-and-white photo showing you the "before" picture, and then the really nice color close-up as the "after" photo. All the celebrity endorsements, or "after" people, are dressed in dark, solid colors because it is more slimming.

I always love to see when they hire a new celebrity to endorse their product. I ask what happened to the other celebrity? In all honesty there are people out there that are born with a wonderful body. Congratulations on winning the genetic lottery. Many people that endorse weight loss products are just that. I want to see the person that was really overweight and transformed their body. That is the person that motivates me. Most people, including myself, need to work at it. It all comes down to discipline, self-control, knowledge, and effort.

I remember growing up in Chicago with the world's best pizza and hot dogs. My dad owned a gas station and would bring home cases of soda. That is what I grew up on.

When I stopped growing as a young kid, I grew the other way. I really put on weight. I had the love handles as free gifts too. My cousins lived across the street and were athletic growing up. Fast forward many years, and I am a doctor that studied physiology and nutrition, and was able to transform my body.

When I say some won the genetic lottery, my cousin had a near perfect physique. He had "it". I am not sure what "it" is, but I know I wanted "it", and the girls want it. But, "it" does not come in a pill, potion, or lotion. The problem with him is that he is a chain smoker and alcoholic. He looks real good on the outside, or at least he did. If you fix the internal environment, it will express outward.

It is funny, or I should say it is sad to me, that people will try these fad diets. I am going to name as many as I can from the top of my head. You can, of course, add to the list. What I do not want you to do, is take this list and go and try them -- the reason, because they do not work. These are fads and gimmicks and are designed to make someone else money.

As a Chiropractor, I get real upset when other health-care professionals, frankly just flat-out lie to their patients, and use scare tactics. This is not a book about Chiropractic or medicine, but there are facts and science, and there is science fiction. As like a good Sci-Fi movie, marketing is key.

My lists of fad diets, in no particular order, are as follows:

Scarsdale diet, caveman diet, grapefruit 45, juicing, Beverly Hills diet, South Beach, Atkins, baby food diet, cabbage soup, HCG, EC Berry diet, three-day diet, Mayo Clinic diet, negative calorie diet, Hollywood diet, apple cider vinegar diet, Sacred Heart diet, etc., etc., etc. How many of those have you heard of before?

I think part of the problem is we have TV shows like *The Biggest Loser*. I have seen only a few minutes of the show. The main problem with it is they always talk about pounds and getting on a scale. You must lose pounds -- pounds, pounds, and pounds. I lost five pounds of fat and gained five pounds of muscle. The scale was the same, but my body was vastly difference. Muscle does not weigh more than fat. I hate when people say that. Muscle is more dense than fat. So the same slice of muscle weighs more than the same slice of fat.

Percentage of body fat is more important than a shrinking scale. I told you to cover up the numbers on your scale, whether it is digital or analog. Get a piece of paper or print out the exact weight that you want to be. If someone wants to weigh 180 pounds, fine. Cover up all the numbers on the scale and write a big 180 and tape it to the top. Every morning when you get up, go on the scale, take a deep breath, close your eyes, and say "I now weigh 180" and looked down and see the 180. I promise you, that alone will help get your mind right. I know that is talking about weight, and I want less body fat. However, this is still a wonderful goal setting technique.

Getting back to some of those big corporations....there is always those oh-so-small words on the bottom of the TV. Do you know what they say? They typically, say something like, "your results may vary" or "results not typical". In fact, you would be shocked to learn the success rate of places like NutriSystem or Jenny Craig. I found those statistics. It is less than one percent. For every 100 people that sign up with NutriSystem or Jenny Craig, 1 out of 100 may get the results.

I am going to comment on a few of the others here. HCG stands for human chorionic gonadotropin. It is still popular today and simply ripping people off from their money.

This HCG is a hormone that is excreted in the urine of pregnant women. What is terrible about this HCG diet is that a lot of doctors sell it and promote it. The major problem with it is that you starve yourself. The protocols for the HCG diet are to eat about 800 calories a day and then get the injection of the "magic potion" and you will keep the weight off. The idea is that you can go ahead and starve yourself (and we talked about this before that your body will go into starvation mode and start using muscle tissue and bone mass for fuel which make you osteoporotic, weaker, and unbalanced). The thought is as long as you get this injection that will not happen. It is completely and utterly false. If you consume only 800 hundred calories per day, you can inject yourself with a liquid Twinkie, and you will lose weight initially. Do not fall for this and waste your money. The fact that you are injecting a hormone, which my guess is synthetic, makes it that much more unsafe.

I have always worked for myself and had my own offices. During a transition of selling an office and buying another one, I worked in a high-volume office with four doctors and about 15 staff members. When you have that many people around, and that many patients, you certainly hear about a lot of different diets. How about the negative calorie diet? The idea behind this is that certain foods, during digestion, would actually burn more calories than were in them themselves. Let us use celery for example. It has been said that celery has negative calories, meaning that the calories of celery, would actually burn more calories. This is not true and completely and utterly false. There are no magical properties or negative calorie foods. A calorie is a measurement. It is like saying a certain log on the fireplace actually burns two logs. The only negative value from anything is ice-cold water. Your body actually has to raise the water temperature and requires energy to do so.

At least some diets discuss fibrous complex carbs, translation -- green vegetables. Green vegetables are very low in calories, and you can eat a ton of them without gaining weight. Every food requires some energy in order to digest it. This is called the thermic effect of food. Talk to any quality trainer that discusses nutrition, and they will say that instead of having a protein shake, to have a lean piece of fish or chicken, etc., because it takes more energy to digest the food than a drink. Many green vegetables have a lot of their calories used up just to digest them. Examples of these are: asparagus, broccoli, cabbage, cauliflower, celery, and zucchini. Fibrous types of vegetables are very filling, very nutritious, and are low in calories.

We have all heard about the Atkins diet, go ahead and eat nothing but protein. The problem with the Atkins diet, is when you consume too much protein, you can actually acidify your body and your blood. We want to move to an alkaline-type of environment for our body for optimal health. The way we accomplish this is with a lot of green vegetables. If you have a lot of lean protein – fish, chicken, meat, etc., and add a lot of green vegetables, you will do very well. Understanding that the Atkins diet is mostly eating protein, no matter what the source, you cannot just order three hot dogs, throw away the buns, and consider that healthy or consider that your weight loss plan.

How about older plans like Deal-a-meal? You have a point value for all foods. Sure, you could have a Big Mac, fries and a Coke, but now you cannot eat anything else for the rest of the day. Like I said before, it is a lot more than calories in and calories out.

If you look at all the marketing lately, it all appears to be starting with "the secret is out". It is not that a secret is out, or that we have discovered some plant in South Africa that has never been touched and all their natives are all lean and muscular. It reminds me of when I was in Chiropractic school. The popular supplement at that time was shark cartilage -- shark cartilage? If you had joint pain or wanted to prevent cancer, apparently you had to get the cartilage of a shark to heal you -- more marketing to make money.

I am not going to go through the list of every fad diet out there, but I am going to mention the one that actually made sense to me, and that was the reverse diet. So if it has some science behind it, then it may offer some benefits. I think a lot of "science" is people taking bits and pieces of a larger puzzle and claiming it as law.

If you look at the typical American diet, it goes like this. Wake up in the morning, skip breakfast and grab some coffee. Lunch is probably fast food consisting of a sandwich with bread, etc. Then for dinner you have some pizza and soda. Dinner is typically your largest meal of the day.

What happens with that typical American diet is the fact that when you wake up, your body has not consumed food for 8 to 12 hours. The fact that you want to skip breakfast, grab a cup of coffee and go -- I promise you by the time you get to work that you will be craving something and maybe eat a bagel or a granola bar. You are putting your body in starvation mode and you are dropping your blood sugar way down. The effect is that around lunchtime you are starving, and even that quick fix, a fast food sandwich, will not last, because by 3 or 4 o'clock, the crash happens again. You are looking for a candy bar to tide you over until you get home and have that really large carb meal.

Try and imagine that scenario reversed. You got up in the morning and had a huge meal. What would happen then, is that since you gave your body something, you would avoid starvation mode. Then typically you would not have any large cravings for carbs because at least you fueled it in the morning. Plus with your first meal of the day being the largest, that means you have all day to burn off those calories. When your last meal of the day is your smallest, your body does not require as much energy to burn off the smaller meal. Of course, I am not suggesting that you have that large pepperoni pizza and Pepsi for breakfast and skip dinner. The point is, its still a fad, but at least it has some merit.

The baby food diet is amazing if you are a stockholder at Gerber. If you are an adult, and you want to eat baby food, you have some serious issues (Jennifer Aniston). By eating smashed carrots, again this is just a super low caloric intake, that will probably work initially, and then your body will compensate. You will get bored with it and will put the weight back on. Sorry, but I would bet that Jennifer Aniston has always been thin. Fad dieters always gain the weight back, and more.

Now, after reading this chapter, someone is going to e-mail me and say that my best friend's cousin's neighbor's buddy lost 50 pounds using HCG or cabbage soup and has kept it off for 10 years -- really? Is that the norm? If that is truly the case, well good for them. There is always the example of the 80 year-old woman that has smoked cigarettes since she was 12 and does not have cancer. Again, is that the norm, or is that just a very rare event? I am telling you science vs. fads.

Please do not fall for these fads or the ads to lose 30 pounds in 30 days. It is impossible. Oh sure, you can talk to any high school wrestling coach and asked them how to make weight. Losing water weight is not hard, and that is what the wrestling coaches do. You can drop water weight, but this is truly not a good idea.

Fads are not limited to diet plans, but also supplements as well. A quick Google search of the top weight loss supplements will reveal the following: Hoodia, Hydroxycut, Trim Spa, CortiSlim, Stacker 2, Alli, and Zantrex. Let us look at a few of these briefly.

Hoodia is an appetite suppressant. That is not an effective way to lose weight and is simply starvation. Hydroxycut's and Trim Spa's main ingredient was ephedra. Ephedra is now banned and both of these products are simply ineffective and unsafe. CortiSlim has Hoodia in it and the main selling point is to reduce cortisol. Cortisol is your stress hormone and can indirectly cause weight gain. Simply by lowering your stress hormone, will not provide any long-lasting benefits or success with weight loss.

The products such as Stacker 2 and Zantrex are nothing more than caffeine-based stimulants in an attempt to increase your metabolism. These two are also not worth the money and are equally ineffective in losing weight.

The last product is Alli, which is a fat blocker. It is, in fact, very effective at blocking fat absorption from the foods you consume. Unfortunately that is not the problem. We need fats in our diet and we need to avoid, again, the process of too many bad carbs which affects insulin and blood sugar levels. Alli is very effective for blocking the absorption of fats in the foods you eat. However, they do need to go somewhere. With this product, your body will become a very effective poop machine. In fact, the makers of the products will tell you to wear dark undergarments to protect potential stains in the very real possibility that you will not be able to control your bowels – oh that sounds nice!

If you do not want to use the big companies or wear brown colored underwear, you can wait on some new technology. The brilliant minds have come up with a pump that is implanted in the body, and after you eat, you flip a switch. (I guess a remote). The pump will remove the contents of the somewhat digested food from your stomach and pump it out of your body. Are you serious? I thought that is called Bulimia? <u>Do not do that!</u> It is always the brain trusts on the medical side that continue to chase symptoms and offer very little in terms of solutions to complex problems.

You must decide to make a commitment to change a little bit of your lifestyle. Did you gain weight overnight? No. Are you going to get rid of it overnight? No. Allow your body to do what it was meant to do, burn mostly fat versus sugar.

Every single one of those fad diets will be replaced by something new, year after year. It will be some fancy catch phrase, some cool new gadget, or something for you to buy. Do me a favor. Let someone else buy it.

One of my Christmas jobs when I was in college was working at UPS. I was a truck loader during the holiday season. Wow, people ship a lot of presents! This was BEFORE companies like Amazon and Internet buying. The number one physique change that people wanted to make, and still is, was to flatten their stomachs. Someone came up with what looked like a small little plastic sled, that was cut in half, that you essentially rocked back and forth on to help your abs. Needless to say, the product did not work, nor did it last very long on the market. However, during my time at UPS, I personally never saw so many of these ab things in my life. Remember, abs are made in the kitchen, not the gym.

Stay away from fads, stay away from quick fixes, and remember things take time. As I tell my patients, be a patient patient. We all want to have instant riches and instant results, but I am telling you, you can get there, if you would just give it a chance.

The fastest way to change is with optimal nutrition and optimal exercise. The next best way is with optimal nutrition. Only when you have great nutrition, you get great results. If you have average results, it is probably from average nutrition. I will give you strategies, so if you decide to accelerate the process by going to the gym, I will show you ways that you can cut your training by more than half and get better results.

To summarize this chapter, please stop looking for a quick fix. Stop searching for the magic pill, potion, or lotion. It does not exist. Apply the science of this book and good things will happen.

Sometimes health restoration is like remodeling a kitchen. You have to remove and demolish the old cabinets, counters, and appliances. The kitchen looks worse. The next thing you know, the new dry wall is up, holes are patched, and fresh paint goes on. It is starting to take shape. Then the new appliances, cabinets, and countertops are in, and you then have a great looking kitchen. Things take time. Life is ups and downs. The secret is to have more ups than downs.

Be well for today and tomorrow.

Chapter 8

Muscles and Aging

In this chapter I am going to talk about muscles. Most of us cannot see ours because layers of fat surround them. Muscles are not just for glamour, they are very important to our physiology and well being.

Did you ever wonder why your grandparents get weaker as they get older? It is not just for the fact that they are older and that is just what happens. It is actually based on their nutrition and loss of muscle mass over the years. Understand this fact. The elderly typically do not die from things like cancer and heart disease. The majority of deaths in elderly people typically follow complications after a broken bone, such as a hip or leg. By improving your muscle mass and tone, you will not only become leaner and healthier, but it can literally save your life.

I am going to discuss the basic functions of muscles along with the different types of muscles. There are what is called type I and type II muscle fibers. These are also known as fast twitch and slow twitch muscle fibers. If you understand how to train them, you can maximize your exercise efforts.

Muscle has high water content and, therefore, is actually much denser than bone. You might be surprised to learn that muscle comprises about 50% of our body weight.

Muscles perform basic functions. First, muscles provide postural support. Muscles provide stability and postural tone to help us stand and hold position. Second, muscles allow us to move and perform work. As they maintain position, they allow protection to our internal organs as well as function. Lastly, muscles are the primary source for generating heat in the body.

Warm-blooded animals have to produce heat to survive or they will die. Obviously, the colder the environment, the more heat they need to generate. Note, if your core body temperature falls below 93°, your heart is likely to stop. If your temperature rises above 108°, proteins in your brain start to break down causing permanent brain damage.

All muscle activity is based on contraction. That is all muscles can do -- contract. Shivering, when the body is cold is produced the same way, by contraction to generate heat. You ever wonder how your limbs extend? Opposing pairs of muscles contracting accomplish all motion. The contraction is initiated by electrical activity. Think of sixth-grade biology, when you dissected a frog. Electrodes were placed on a certain position and made the leg muscles fire and the frog contract its leg.

There are three types of muscles in the body: smooth muscle, cardiac muscle, and skeletal muscle. Smooth muscle is a type of muscle that is found in the arteries, veins, bladder, uterus, male and female reproductive tracts, gastrointestinal tract, and respiratory tract. Smooth muscle is different from skeletal muscle in terms of function and mechanism of contraction.

Cardiac muscle is found in the walls of the heart. Its contractions propel blood both into the heart and then through the arteries of the circulatory system. Unlike skeletal muscle, these contractions are primarily involuntary.

Skeletal muscle is the muscle that I want to discuss. It is similar to cardiac muscle but it has different characteristics and uses. Skeletal muscle is found attached to bone, skin, fascia, and other muscles. The main difference is that skeletal muscles are voluntary. This means that the contractions of the skeletal muscles happen when we choose to make them happen. Like when we lift our arms. Cardiac and smooth muscle, as discussed, are primarily involuntary. Your heart will beat whether you think about it or not.

Muscle contractions happen at the smallest level with two proteins. The thick filament is made of the protein myosin, and the thin filament is made from the protein actin. That is why protein consumption is important in muscle development and is necessary. Protein is the fundamental building block in muscle. Essentially, these muscles get triggered by a nerve impulse and then the muscle contracts.

To build muscle and create a leaner physique, you need several things. First is protein. Muscle is built from protein. You obviously need protein to build muscle. However, if you are not doing extreme levels of exercise, then you do not need massive amounts of protein. You need HGH. Your body produces HGH or human growth hormone. I will tell you ways that you can get your body to release HGH naturally. You do not want to take HGH injections or something artificial.

While building muscle and maintaining muscle, you also need plenty of hydration. So many people do not drink enough water. By avoiding water and putting foods in our body that dehydrate us, such as caffeine, we are setting ourselves up for muscle weakness, fatigue, and injury. Muscles need to be able to slide and glide over themselves, just like your joints. It is necessary for you to drink plenty of water every day. How much water you need is based on your size. Forget the common 8, 8oz glasses per day. You can drink a third, to up to a half, of your body weight in ounces of water. A 200-pound person can drink 100 ounces of water per day.

If you are interested in making sure your muscles fire, then you need to do everything to allow for proper nerve flow. Omega 3 fatty acids are a requirement, which are commonly found in fish and fish oil supplements, and are a necessary component in your daily needs. Vitamin D also helps to protect from demyelination of the nerves. Toxic heavy metals accumulation can also affect nerve impulses. A heavy metal detox once or twice per year is essential for optimal health. I recommend using jonbarron.org for any detox program you choose.

When I discuss energy for the muscles, I recommend that every adult be on enzyme CoQ10. In fact, statin drugs, which are used for lowering cholesterol, suppress the liver's synthesis of cholesterol. These drugs tell the liver do not make as much cholesterol. The same pathway in which that occurs also suppresses and blocks CoQ10. If you are on a statin drug, you must supplement with CoQ10. It is also a good supplement for your heart, as is omega 3 fatty acids.

I recommend that everybody take those supplements. I never recommend the use of statin drugs. They have tremendous side effects. Essentially they may be good for the pipes, but not so much for the pump.

Muscles will begin to break down at some point. Some studies suggest it is 30 years of age. I will tell you that our muscle mass can begin to decrease in our late 20s. I tell my patients that we hit a fork in the road at around the age of 35, plus or minus a few years, based on your health.

A person can lose about 1% of their muscle mass each year after the age of 30. After the age of 50, the rate in which we lose muscle mass is accelerated. We need muscle for our protection as well as for the function of our internal chemistry. When we do not feed our bodies with what it needs, our bodies will begin to break down. You must be consciously aware that your muscles are not just something pretty to look at. They are supporting our skeleton, they are supporting our spine, and they are protecting our internal organs. Think of muscles as soldiers surrounding your property. The more soldiers you have, the better protection you have. Try to imagine that every year, fewer soldiers are protecting your house. Eventually you are going to have your property wide open for a massive takeover from the bad guys.

By choosing better nutrition and increasing your lean protein consumption, balanced with green vegetables, you can not only slow this process way down, but in some cases reverse a portion of it.

Take a look at the statistics. Muscle loss starts at .5% to 2% per year. This number can accelerate based on your age, nutritional habits, and as well as your exercise habits. The loss of muscle mass is called sarcopenia. Over the course of your life, and into your 70s, you can lose a total of 45% of your muscle mass.

When I am discussing muscle mass loss, I am discussing degeneration. There are other conditions that can cause muscle loss from diseases, and also some medications which can induce muscle loss. The main problem with muscle loss is it can affect our balance and something called proprioception. Proprioception is our body's awareness of its position. For example, if you close your eyes and I extend your fingers, you would realize it was pointing up or down. That is proprioception.

When it comes to muscles, there is a saying you should become well aware of, "use it or lose it." Nothing could be more accurate in that statement. This book is about nutrition. Poor nutrition, such as too much sugar and processed foods, combined with a lack of protein, will decrease your muscle mass. With lack of protein, your muscles cannot regenerate. The sad part is when you lose muscle mass, it is replaced with fat.

Even a neurological disease such as Guillain Barre Syndrome can be attributed with muscle loss. By increasing your muscle mass with proper nutrition and adequate amounts of protein, your body will be better protected and you will have better internal chemistry.

Being a Chiropractor for over 15 years, I have developed a lot of patterns and similarities with patients. The magic age that I tell patients is 35. Again, this is plus or minus five years. Make sure, regardless of your age, that you be aware of your muscle mass and be conscious that you need to fuel the body and not just feed the body.

So many people today are electing for HRT, which is hormone replacement therapy. Again, that is your choice, but I do not recommend artificially changing your chemistry when it can self-regulate with proper nutrition.

I will tell you, as a Chiropractor, most people go to the medical doctor and received medications or received injections for pain, prior to seeing me. Too many of these injections can actually weaken the soft tissues and set the patient up for a future surgery. Most neck and back surgeries can be avoided and should be. The point is, the body is the most amazing machine ever. It has a tremendous ability to heal and repair itself, if you do the proper things. Disrespect and neglect your health and it will catch up with you. It is your body and your health.

By adding adequate amounts of lean protein, avoiding processed foods and sugar, and incorporating a weightlifting program at any age, can slow down Father Time. Sadly, there is nothing we can do about slowing down time. In my office, we say "it is your future, be there healthy".

Let us talk a little bit more about aging and muscle mass. As I have mentioned, we can lose anywhere from .5% to 1%, sometimes even 2%, of our muscle mass per year from our mid-30s, 40s, and 50s and so on. So, let us use the age of 35, and say that it is 1% each year, that is 5% every 10 years. It may not sound like a lot, but it is a tremendous amount when you look at the implications of living your life with less muscle mass. The human body is an amazing adaptive organism. It fights for survival every day or it dies. Heart disease, diabetes, and weight gain can all be reversed if you take the time and do what is right for your body.

One main problem that we have in this country, is the fact that too many people are eating too much of the wrong stuff, loaded with chemicals, and are drinking too many sugary calories. When the body breaks down, they further pollute it with medications. Your health is in your hands. Do not let anyone let you believe otherwise. If you want to live on medications and spend your day going from doctor to doctor, then that is your business. I prefer to take a pro-active approach to my health and well-being.

Understand, I am not anti-medicine or anti-surgery. I am saying that too many people just do not take the responsibility and the effort for their own health. When the body breaks down, they run out for a pill or a shot. Remember, you are running the greatest corporation known, your health, treat it as such, and take more responsibility for it.

Historically, our bodies were designed as hunters and gatherers, to be strong and fit, and around until the age of about 35. From there, a younger generation would take over the responsibility. Our most difficult time today in getting food is being the fourth car in line at the drive thru.

It seems that our bodies still follow a similar pattern. Around the age of 35 we really start to accelerate muscle mass loss. The main problem is when we lose muscle we typically replace it with fat. In order to retain our current weight as we reach middle age, we need to lower our caloric intake by anywhere between 150 and 450 calories per day.

The other option is to work hard on building muscle mass to avoid this fat gain. By applying more protein to our daily diet, we can avoid the dreaded "muffin top" as we age.

Lean body mass consists of biologically active tissue that includes: muscle, bone, nerve, and vital organ tissue. All of these have a greater calorie burning capacity than fat. When we lose lean body mass, we sadly, and unfortunately, loose the most active of all tissues. This changes our metabolism, and slows it way down. The fact that our metabolism slows as we age creates a double-edged sword. The loss of lean body tissue produces a loss of muscle strength and accelerates as we age. With the combined loss of muscle strength and power, it will eventually lead to a greater difficulty in performing your daily activities. This will then increase the chances of injuring yourself.

Older bodies are less efficient at building muscle than younger ones. Also note, blood flow to the legs also decreases with age, depriving the muscle of nutrients. Numerous studies will point out that increasing activity, and consuming more lean proteins, will improve not only muscle mass, but also circulation to the lower extremities. In fact, much of the muscle weakness was completely reversed.

Lean proteins need to be consumed <u>at each meal</u>, examples are: eggs, lean meats, fish, cottage cheese, etc. This provides the body with the building blocks necessary to build muscle. Adequate restful sleep is also required. It is never too late to build muscle mass at any age. This will help with more endurance, improved flexibility, and general overall health. Do not confuse the term "mass" with looking like a massive body builder. We are talking about adding muscle tissue.

In my Insulin chapter, I talked about insulin and the responses of insulin, with a rapid rise in blood sugar, based on high carbs or sugary foods. Insulin drives amino acids, which are the building blocks of proteins, into our muscles. Muscles respond to insulin much differently in a 25 year-old male versus a 60 year-old male. Therefore, age does limit muscles from responding to insulin and, therefore, can even prevent the muscles from taking in more amino acids to build muscle. It is much easier for a young person to add muscle to his/her physique versus a older person.

Muscles loose size and strength as we get older, which will contribute to fatigue and weakness. Muscle fibers, themselves, are reduced in their number and shrink as we age. Muscle tissue is replaced more slowly, and lost muscle tissue is replaced with more of a rough fibrous tissue.

The fact that most people do not utilize my incredible profession of Chiropractic to get their spine adjusted creates in them a lack of spinal motion, which affects nerve flow, and nerves fire the muscles. By avoiding and neglecting the spine, you can actually have weaker muscles. I recommend everybody find a Chiropractor and get their spines adjusted on a regular basis. When patients get their lower cervical spine (neck) adjusted, it stimulates the thyroid gland and, therefore, stimulates their metabolism to speed up. They sleep better and, consequently, the side effects are more energy and weight loss.

If your body is deficient in some nutrients, your body will not function as well. I think that is obvious. You must eat a lot of protein to keep your muscles from shrinking. This is why people trying to lose fat, without sacrificing muscle, do best when they build their nutrition around high- quality protein from lean meat, fish, eggs, and poultry.

Protein has qualities that help weight loss and can prevent weight gain. Protein is metabolically expensive for your body to process. Your body burns about 20% of each protein calorie just in digesting it. Protein creates a high level of satiety. In other words, you feel fuller faster, and it keeps you feeling fuller longer between meals. Like anything with your body, it can become accustomed to it and will adapt. Just like consuming a lot of water. If you are not someone who consumes a lot of water, you will be going to the bathroom a lot. Eventually your body will adjust to that.

You can categorize this under the law of diminishing returns. What that means is anything that goes in your body for a long period of time will eventually not be as effective. If you are a coffee drinker that needs a caffeine boost, after about 30 to 60 days, your body will adjust and regulate from caffeine. Your body will adjust. Those of you who are getting a "boost" from caffeine, it is because your body has actually fallen below the level it would have been at without caffeine. Caffeine will bring you up to a level just below where you would have been without it. It is no different from using melatonin to fall asleep or any medication that you may be taking.

Getting back to protein, if you eat more protein than your body needs, it will learn to use the protein for energy. You want your body to burn carbs and fat for energy. You want your body to burn the fat for fuel. The point is to not overdo your protein. It would be like your car engine using its engine parts for fuel versus the gasoline.

What amount do you need? Some will say that you should have 2g of protein per kilogram of body weight. A kilogram is 2.2 pounds. You can look at 70% to 80% of your weight in grams of protein. Trust me, it is a lot of protein and it is difficult to consume that much if you are not used to it. In my opinion, it will take you several weeks to increase your protein and regulate your blood sugar so you are not having blood sugar spikes.

When you make your protein choices, make sure that you are making quality choices. You cannot go to McDonald's, throw the bun away, and just eat the meat or whatever they call it. Lean proteins are what the body needs. Let me tell you quickly that if you are concerned with eggs and cholesterol, do not be. Cholesterol is the biggest myth out there. Eating an egg yolk is perfectly healthy for you. The yolk has a lot of amino acids. You want to buy organic, free-range eggs whenever possible.

At the end of the book, I will give you an Action Plan for the first two weeks and then slowly introduce a little carbs. This is not some Atkins diet.

Guess what? You can do it. Again, the definition of insanity is "doing the same thing over and over again and expecting different results". Get out of your comfort zone. Do not look at it as something you are forced to do. Look at it as something you want to do.

You can always go back, McDonald's and Pepsi are not going anywhere (if that is your thing). Life is about the journey, not the destination. Set short-term goals that feed into your long-term goals.

I look at my children. I have three boys. At the time of writing this book, their ages are 11, 9 and 5. The 11 year-old is in sixth grade, the 9 year-old is in fourth grade, and the 5 year-old is in preschool. My 11 year-old looks at everything as an exciting opportunity, a challenge, and it is going to be great. He, of course, was nervous about middle school, but looked at it that he will make new friends and can play sports for the school. My 9 year-old looks at many things as a chore and a task. He puts a lot of stress on himself and drags his feet a lot. My point here is very clearly, look at this book as an opportunity of creating an all new you.

You see yourself every day. Others in your life may not see you for three months, six months, or even a year. This is what motivates me. I see my best friend twice a year. I look forward to getting off that plane, walking into his house, and for him to say, "Wow, you look good!"

For me it is exciting to experiment with protein and cut out the carbs. It is exciting for me, because I now look at things as a gift and a lesson. Being a Chiropractor can be the most frustrating thing in my life. People say, find a job you love and you will never have to go to work. I love Chiropractic! It's awesome! I have helped so many people over the years with just my two hands and my knowledge. What I do not like about my profession sometimes, is people. Let me explain. Chiropractic works just about every time. What does not work, is people and their compliance to a treatment plan. The same is for this book. The information in here works. It is science based. What may not work is your adherence to the plan.

If all these new diet books that come out every year get you excited to do something, then great! If they all worked, there would not be a need for another new book. <u>The point is, it is all about compliance. The magic word that you should learn is discipline. Just a little bit goes a long way</u>.

As you read this book, please just start to do "something". For everyone that reads this book, let us look at the bell curve. Ten percent will read the book and never do a darn thing. Another 10% will do everything in this book to the letter. The majority of the people will start to do a little bit, get excited, stop for a while, maybe go back and try it again. At the end of this book, when you get to the plan portion, I will discuss, what I call, the 2-1-2 plan that will make compliance easier.

Let me give you a real world example. A good friend of mine and I were hanging out. This person is not very healthy. He lives on diet soda, beer, and a lot of processed foods. Add in a highly stressful job, lack of sleep, and you have a person that is overweight and unhealthy. Right around the time of the New Year he was going to make some changes. His plan was to buy some fat blocking supplements. I did not say a word, nor did he ask me my opinion. If he did I would have discouraged him. At this point, if you think that fat is the problem, then you have not been reading this book. Too many calories, too many empty calories, and bad food choices are the problem. So this is the big reason I did not say anything. Let us say he goes out and buys this supplement. Maybe, the pill helps him consciously with his food choices, and he loses five pounds. Even if it is water weight, or whatever, it may be enough to make him feel better, and now he wants to improve even further. If 5 pounds turns into 10 pounds, and losing 10 pounds turns into a gym membership. The gym membership turns into healthier eating choices, and this is great. So I would never discourage somebody from doing something that MAY be the start of a healthier lifestyle.

My Chiropractic office sits next to two medical offices. The medical office next to my office sells and promotes HCG injections (I do not feel it offers any real solution). When I had a few of my patients tell me that they went over there to do it, I said great, go for it. I never said it was a scam to them, nor did I say do not do it. Again, it might be the catalyst that gets them moving in the right direction. If I felt something was unsafe and dangerous, then I will point that out.

In the case of one of my most recent patients, the HCG injection did not work in the slightest. She was quite overweight when she started. By greatly reducing her calories for two weeks, she lost pounds. After about three weeks of essentially starving herself, she went back to her normal routine and put all the weight back on, and then some. This is what happens with crash and fad diets.

I have another patient who is 35, divorced, and really felt compelled to get into great physical shape as she was now "back on the market." Her words, not mine. She tells me of the hours and hours of exercise that she puts in daily. She goes to a trainer where she works out with weights for about 45 minutes every day. At the end of her day she gets on her elliptical for another 45 minutes. You would think with all of this exercise that this woman would be in amazing shape. Guess what? She is not. Two reasons, she is not training correctly, and her nutritional intake is way too low. As a result of this increased activity, without the proper fuel, she is tired, lethargic, and not losing the weight that she wants.

To summarize this chapter, you must eat correctly, with plenty of protein. You have to eat often. You can reward yourself with any type of food. I promise that you will still enjoy anything you want. I will get you to that point.

It is your health and your future health. Remember, nothing tastes as good as thin feels.

Chapter 9

Acid vs. Alkaline

In this chapter, I want to discuss the importance of alkalizing your blood and your body. There are a lot of companies out there that are selling water purification systems that will offer to alkaline your water. Other companies sell drops that you can add to your water to make it more alkaline. Tremendous amounts of health claims are made saying, that by just drinking alkaline-based water, your body is going to heal and cure itself from a wide range of symptoms and ailments.

You can achieve the same thing by having a proper diet. There is nothing wrong with adding a little alkalinity to your water, but I do not think it is a cure-all. But heck, there are a lot of worse things that you can do for your health. So I say go for it. You just do not need go out and spend hundreds, or even thousands, of dollars on a machine. There are several herbalists and vitamin shops in my town that offer alkaline water to their customers. Bring in a few containers and then fill them up.

So why is this important and what does this mean? Simply put, if you live in the United States of America, your diet is very acidic. So when I talk about acidity and alkalinity, we have to go back to junior high school and remember the pH scale of acids and bases.

Our pH is a measure of exactly how acidic or alkaline we are. The range on the pH scale is 0 to 14. A pH of 0 is completely acidic, while a pH of 14 is completely alkaline or basic. A pH of 7 is considered neutral. Your body does not have one pH level. It has more than one, and has ranges. Just like for blood pressure, people gravitate towards 120/80, or a body temperature of 98.6°. These are averages, when, in fact, there are ranges of healthy levels of blood pressure or body temperature.

Your stomach has a pH ranging from 1.3 to 3.5. It must be acidic to aid in the digestion of food. However, our blood must always be slightly alkaline with a pH of around 7.35 – 7.45. The idea of an alkaline-based diet, or alkaline water, is that eating certain foods can help maintain the body's ideal pH to improve overall health. The body will maintain its pH balance regardless of diet.

As I mentioned, your blood pH should be slightly alkaline. If you are below or above this range, it typically results in symptoms and disease. An acidic pH can occur from an acid forming diet, emotional stress, toxic overload, or any process that deprives the cells of oxygen and other nutrients. The body will try to compensate for acidic pH by using alkaline minerals from your body. If your diet does not contain enough minerals to compensate, a buildup of acids in the cells will occur.

An acidic balance will decrease the body's ability to absorb minerals and other nutrients, decrease the energy production in the cells, decrease its ability to repair damaged cells, decrease its ability to detoxify heavy metals, make tumor cells arrive, and make you more susceptible to fatigue and illness. A blood pH of 6.9, which is only slightly acidic, can induce coma and death.

The reason acidosis is more common in our society, is mostly due to the typical American diet also known as the Standard American Diet (S.A.D.). Of course, we can just call it SAD. The typical American diet is too high in processed foods, and too low in fresh vegetables. When you add in things like white flour, sugar, soft drinks, milk, and coffee, we are creating more acidity in our bodies. Our society uses too many medications (prescription or over-the-counter) and we use artificial sweeteners, like NutraSweet and Splenda, which are poison and extremely acid forming. One of the best things to do to correct an overly acidic body is to clean up the diet and lifestyle.

To <u>maintain</u> one's health, a general rule is that your diet should consist of 60% of alkaline forming foods and 40% of acid forming foods. To <u>restore</u> health, the diet should consist of 80% alkaline forming foods and 20% acid forming foods.

You can do an internet search and find a whole list of alkaline/acid forming foods. Generally, alkaline forming foods include most fruits, green vegetables, peas, beans, lentils spices, herbs, seeds, and nuts. Acid forming foods include most foods that have been processed. I am recommending that people consume a lot of extra protein. Acid forming foods include meat, fish, poultry, and eggs. To neutralize this, have vegetables, specifically green vegetables, with every meal.

Remember that an acidic body is a sickness magnet. Is it any wonder that people that you know, maybe including yourself, are often sick or in pain? When the temperature drops in fall and winter, they "get" everything. My kids, my wife, and I are almost never sick, and if we are, it is always VERY minor. Good nutrition is the main reason. We include exercise and regular chiropractic care, and there you have our recipe for great health!

It is interesting to note that researchers conclude that an alkaline-based diet can slow bone loss and muscle wasting. It can also increase growth hormone, make certain chronic diseases less likely, and ease low back pain.

Further clinical studies have proven that people who eat more fresh fruits and vegetables, and drink plenty of water, do have lower rates of cancer and other diseases.

Many times we talk about health, nutrition, or exercise and there always seems to be some researchers that grab bits and pieces of science and turn it into law. What I mean by that is, for example, someone decides they want to flatten their stomach. So they find out that doing some exercises, like a sit up or a plank, is recommended to improve their core, so that is all they do. Factor in a bunch of late-night infomercials, with a rocker or roller for the abs that focus on the core, and they sell you a junky plastic widget, and there is your secret to a flatter stomach.

A few years ago, it became understood that when your body is stressed, you produce more of a hormone called cortisol. This stress hormone can actually make you gain weight. Well, manufacturers decided to create a supplement that reduces the cortisol and, therefore, problem solved. Unfortunately, the body is much more complex than that. If you want a flatter stomach, and want to see your abs, remember, they are made in the kitchen, not the gym.

Understand that the human body is a very complex machine. It requires regular maintenance. The body is a self-healing, self-regulating machine. Providing your body with what it needs and keeping it more alkaline vs. acidic is what is vital to your health. Increasing your vitamin D will really help you stay healthy. If you cannot get 15 minutes of daily sunlight, then supplementation can help with your Vitamin D intake.

So as the human body is constantly regulating, if you are a regular user of caffeinated products, your body has to adjust to that stimulus. Many people feel they cannot start the day without caffeine. This will create more acidity in the body. Eating an apple in the morning can give you more energy than a cup of coffee.

What happens is that your internal chemistry must stay in balance through alkalization? How will this affect your bone health? It will hurt it. Do you know what I call diet soda? Liquid osteoporosis. It is a horrible beverage choice. I am so surprised that people actually drink diet soda. First of all it, tastes gross, and is loaded with artificial sweeteners. If you want a soda, then drink one. Of course, high fructose corn syrup has caused more obesity than probably any other product on earth. Look at the people that drink diet soda on a regular basis, most of them are obese. Drink your water!

So why is diet soda osteoporosis in a can? Though most of our tissues are alkaline in nature, digesting certain foods, and even breathing, creates acid that needs neutralizing. The body can neutralize some per day without going into the alkaline reserves stored in our bones. Sadly, the diet that most people in the U.S. eat every day produces about double of what the body can handle.

This means, that on a daily basis, our bodies have to use mineral compounds that make up our bones to neutralize the over abundance of acid in our bodies. So I guess if you want weak bones, sickness, disease, and obesity, and want to be a typical American, then make no changes in your life -- toss this book away, go hit the drive-thru, and enjoy yourself.

So how do you get more alkalinity in your life? By doing more of the same of what I have been talking about. Eat more veggies and fruit. Most plant foods contain an abundance of alkaline particles and create a naturally occurring alkaline balance in your body. Refer to the rule from above, do you need to <u>maintain</u> your health or do you need to <u>restore</u> your health?

You must reduce, but I would say to eliminate, all soft drinks from your diet. This includes regular soda, diet soda, Gatorade, and all of those worthless energy drinks. The main ingredient in any soda is phosphoric acid. This requires your body to sacrifice a great deal of alkalinity from buffering salts and minerals in the bones. Make it easier, just do not do it.

Get rid of all your processed carbs. You can eventually earn a few carbs in your diet, but for now it is a no. You can eat things like sweet potatoes, yams, potatoes, beets, carrots, squash as they are all rich in minerals. So try substituting these items instead of pasta, pizza, pastries, and bread.

You should add fresh lemon or lime to your water. Also, if you like the taste, many people are adding cucumber slices to their water. So help balance your acid load by squeezing a wedge of fresh lemon, lime, or cucumber into your water throughout the day. You can also squeeze a lime on your food or salads before you eat.

Drink water every day. Try and avoid regular tap water unless it is filtered. Most of our public drinking water has chlorine and fluoride levels added that are not healthy for us. You could have high mineral spring water. These include calcium, magnesium, and potassium salts, which will help your alkaline reserves.

Also try adding cinnamon, ginger, and other herbs and spices to your food as well. Cinnamon is a wonderful alkalizing spice that you can add to just about anything. It is great with sweet potatoes, apples, or hot tea. Ginger root is also a great alkalizer and a detoxifier. My favorite spice to add is called Tumeric.

You can monitor your pH by tracking your first morning urine. It is a simple and convenient way to know how your nutritional changes are affecting your body. This number should be between 6.5 and 7.5. Just do a quick Google search and you will see many places you can buy a home Ph test kit, or check my resource page at the end of this book.

I will mention one last thing about pH and blood. Being a doctor has afforded me the benefit of interacting with a lot of people, while helping a lot of patients. Not everybody has a Chiropractor that they use on a regular basis, but everyone has a primary medical doctor that they use. Many times patients will come to me and I will ask to see their blood work. Many times they say, well they tested me, and everything is normal or within normal ranges.

Many times something has to be in your body for a really long time before it shows up on a blood test. There are markers for acute conditions, but for the most part, small subtle changes may not show up in the blood. We call that sub-clinical. It means there are really no obvious signs of something that is occurring, but that does not mean that it is not happening.

Every cell functions optimally within a certain pH range. In different cells, the range is different, however, the net pH of the body has remained tightly regulated. One common problem with most industrialized societies is that our diets produce what is called a low-grade chronic metabolic acidosis. While there are a number of diseases that induce severe metabolic acidosis, I am talking about a sub-clinical rise. Therefore, your medical doctor may not notice the problem.

Here are some of the most severe consequences of your body's attempt to maintain a constant pH in the face of an acidic environment: hypercalciuria is high concentrations of calcium in the urine. Since calcium is a strong base and bone contains the body's largest calcium store, too much acidity causes a release of calcium from the bones. As a result, osteoclasts, which are the bones recyclers, increase their activity while the bone builders, osteoblasts, decrease their activity. The net result is that the bone is lost in order to neutralize the acidic environment of the body.

This creates a negative nitrogen balance. When you have a negative nitrogen balance that means your muscles are breaking down. In life you are either growing or dying.

In addition to lose losing calcium and muscle, other problems or conditions can occur like hypothyroidism and hyper-cortisolemia. By employing a few simple acid based strategies, it can help slow down osteoporosis and sarcopenia (muscle loss).

By making better food choices, and by avoiding poor food choices, not only will you lose weight, but you are actually on the road to becoming healthier. It comes down to a matter of how often you think about your health and future health. How much respect do you have for your body and can you discipline yourself to <u>fuel</u> the body versus <u>feed</u> the body.

I honestly think it is the way that you look at things. Years ago, I purchased this certain supplement -- we are talking 15 years ago -- I think the supplement today is better researched and actually tastes better. But, I used to drink this green drink to alkaline my body, and I took a product designed to detox and cleanse my body. Now, it tasted like wet sand mixed with crackers. It had no taste, and it was actually really gross. It was like a cross between grass clippings and something your dog would throw up. However, I looked at these products as something that was helping my body. By doing so, it took me a very short time to get used to them and actually enjoy them.

I will tell you that I am a former soda-holic, back in the day when it was actually made with real sugar. My dad used to own a gas station. He would bring home cases of soda. That was my staple drink for every meal. Now, it is easier to get off soda than you think. I did not say it was easy, it is just easier than you think.

When I was a young man and my joints started hurting me, I decided I cannot drink this crap anymore. After about two weeks, I was completely off soda, and that has lasted to this day. Now, sometimes I will be at a restaurant having some fun food and I may order a soda. But, the greatest thing is, when you are healthy, your body will absolutely reject it. It simply does not taste good. When you start craving broccoli you know you are a healthy eater.

My soda order is about once every two or three months. I would take a sip and say and realize that this is disgusting. My friends, who are not as healthy as I am, would taste it and tell me that there is nothing wrong with it. The point I am trying to make to you is that you can change your taste buds and re-train your brain to love great healthy foods and reject the junk. It is a matter of being patient and having a little discipline.

Please do not look at these changes in your life as something that you are forced to do. You <u>need</u> to look at them as something that you <u>want</u> to do. You need to tell yourself that you are going to do them. For me to be a Chiropractor and see patients for years has been the biggest "blessing" in my life. Why is that? It is because I have seen young people, to middle-aged people, age incredibly fast with my own eyes, and I know I do not want that.

Two examples come to mind: One person that was in a professional referral group of mine has his own painting business. This is a man that when I met him was in his early 50s. He was a little overweight, a little unhealthy and had no exercise is life. I am not judging this person as I do not know him personally. But, about 18 months later, I contacted him to paint my office, I did not recognize him when he came in for the estimate. I do not feel 18 months is a long time to look completely old and broken down. Health can take a turn - fast. He rode the wave too long of being unhealthy and it caught up with him.

The second example is a patient of mine that would come in sporadically. When it came to following my treatment plan and recommendations, she did not follow them. As a result, she came in a few times, but decided that she was best served with injections and medications. I have personally never seen someone gain so much weight in such a short period of time. She was an attractive woman in her late 30s. But when, she came back to my office about six months later, she had gained 55 pounds. I do not think I could do that unless I drank a 2-liter of soda every day and hit every drive thru for breakfast, lunch, and dinner. I was stunned by her physical appearance. Now understand, that she had some physical pain that she chose to cover up the symptoms with medication. And she also had emotional pain, which she treated with comfort food, which is very common.

The point of these two examples is the fact that this is YOUR life. This is YOUR health. It is not mine, it YOURS. For those of you that have kids, realize how fast they grow up. It seems that once the process of going downhill has started, for many of you, it is the beginning of the end. I see my patients that are 60 years old and retired, spending their days going to different doctors. I do not understand that.

You make choices every day. You must decide what you are going to do with your health. Without health, there is no job for you to go to. Without health, there are no family and friends to hang out with. Without health, there are no activities that you love to do.

I am trying to give you some information on how to become healthier and lose weight without wasting your time at the gym. You have to want it. I would rather you make small changes now, versus some healthcare professional telling you "do this now or die". To me, it is really that simple.

Many of you will read this book and brush it aside and say there was nothing in here I did not know -- really? Then why are you not doing it? What is the reason? That is for you to answer, not me. In life, when your WHY is big enough, you will determine the HOW. Make small choices and set goals. Set short-term goals that lead to a grand long-term goal.

The company Nike still has the greatest slogan – "just do it". You can still enjoy life and enjoy fun foods. When you abide by these rules, you can enjoy more foods, and have a greater ability to enjoy the things in your life. Try this for 90 days. Give it a shot to the best of your ability. The lifestyle you have now will still be there -- choices, choices, and choices.

If you want to spend your life going to the doctors, being sick, taking medication, getting injections, having potential surgeries, then do not change a darn thing. Tell me you eat junk and do not go to the doctors. That may be true. Again, is that the exception or the rule? And, has it just not caught up with you yet?

Roll the dice and see if you can roll the lucky number. If you continue to act like a typical American, then I am putting all my chips on S.A.D. The Standard American Diet is failing this country and also the world. <u>When other countries sell American foods, they start getting American diseases – FACT!</u>

To summarize this chapter, it is important that you understand that your body is in a constant struggle to remain in balance. If you continue to tip the scales the wrong way, understand that you may be accelerating poor health and serious health problems, which are typically handled with drugs, which may also further deplete your internal balance.

Most people truly want to lose weight and become healthier. If this is you, then do it. Two steps forward, and one step back, is still forward. Do it to the best of your ability and be proud of your accomplishments.

It is your health! Be well.

Chapter 10

Metabolism & Tips

The metabolism is that thing that everybody wants to increase. The idea is that it is the secret to weight loss -- just turn up the speed, and you are good to go. Kids have a fast metabolism. They are growing every day. My three boys are hungry every three hours, heck probably every hour. They eat and have a tremendous amount of energy. So what is this thing called metabolism?

Metabolism is from the Greek word, meaning change. Metabolism is the set of chemical transformations within the cells of living organisms that sustain life. These enzyme reactions allow organisms to grow and reproduce, maintain the structures, and respond to their environments. The word itself can also include digestion and the transport of substances into and between different cells.

It seems everyone is selling some sort of metabolism booster to lose weight. I do not recommend most of them, they are mostly made with just caffeine. At the end of this book I am going to give a summary, along with the plan and action steps that you need to do to be totally serious about losing weight. A good friend of mine breaks every one of these rules and, therefore, he is overweight. He loves to spend his money at the vitamin stores, buying the magic fat burners. It has already caught up with him, but he is getting worse with his health. More symptoms and pains are cropping up here and there.

Years ago, there was a program for sale talking about how, when you eat you rev your metabolism, therefore, just go ahead and eat since you are increasing your metabolism. I think the program was called, "You Gotta Eat!" Of course, when you eat, your body requires energy to break down the food. I discussed this in earlier chapters called the thermic effect of food. Just because you are eating does not necessarily mean you are getting a sustained metabolism boost that will cause you to burn fat.

Metabolism is divided into two categories. The two categories are catabolic and anabolic. When you hear the word anabolic, think of anabolic steroids, they build muscles. Catabolic is the opposite; it is a breakdown of muscles and muscle tissue.

The reactions of metabolism are organized into pathways in which one chemical is transformed through a series of steps into another chemical by a sequence of enzymes. Enzymes are crucial to metabolism, because they allow organisms to drive desirable reactions that require energy, which will not occur by themselves, but by coupling them to spontaneous reactions they release energy. As enzymes act as catalysts, they allow these reactions to proceed quickly and efficiently. The metabolism of an organism determines which substances it will find nutritious and poisonous.

While you do not really have much control over the speed of your metabolism, you can control your burn through your level of physical activity and by keeping your body well fed every several hours. Obviously, the more active you are, the more calories you can burn. In fact, some people who are said to have a fast metabolism are probably just more active than others or eat more often. Sometimes it is truly better to graze throughout the day. About every three hours is about the right time for most people.

There really is no magic to increasing your metabolism. Products that claim to speed up your metabolism are often more hype than help, often with dangerous side effects.

Other factors determine your individual basal metabolic rate, which include your body size and composition. The bodies of people who are larger or have more muscle mass, burn more calories at rest. Your sex plays a role too. Men usually have less body fat and more muscle than women do of the same age, therefore, by increasing your muscle mass you can burn more calories at rest. Age is a factor also. As we get older we lose muscle mass, which is then replaced by fat. The less muscle mass you have, the slower your metabolism.

This all goes back to nutrition, nutrition, and nutrition. See how the puzzle pieces are coming together?

You can estimate your basal metabolic rate by Googling a BMI calculator. I prefer you do a Google search for the Harris – Benedict equation. Your basal metabolic rate accounts for 60% to 75% of the calories you burn every day. It gives you an estimate of what your body burns at rest. It does not take into account muscle mass. I want you to do that to get an idea so that if you have limited activity, and you consume say 2000 calories per day, many of you, unfortunately, will recognize that you are getting that with one meal. I am not asking you to count calories. If you consume mostly lean protein and vegetables, you will never have to. I just want you to see how fast stuff adds up.

In addition to physical activity and lifestyle choices, the processing of food accounts for about 10% of the calories used each day. This includes digestion, absorbing, transporting, and storing the food you consume.

This is a good time to assume that, if you are overweight, you will want to blame your metabolism. I have a slow metabolism and, therefore, that is why. My comment to that is -- please stop making excuses. Do you want reasons or results? Go to my website, NOGYMGOSLIM.com to stay motivated.

Understand that metabolism is a natural process in your body and will balance to meet your individual needs. As I have said, the body is a self-healing, self-regulating organism. It will adapt. This is the reason why if you try these very restrictive diets, your body will compensate by slowing down. Your machine, known as your body, will slow down those processes and conserve your calories for survival. Extreme restriction of calories can result in your body using muscle mass or bone tissue as an energy source. Eventually, when you do go back to a more normal routine, you will actually put on more weight than you started with. This is the pattern of yo-yo dieting.

This is why I said I was strongly against fad diets and things like the HCG diet. The bottom line is, weight gain is the process of one eating too many calories, eating too fast, and creating an insulin response that spikes blood sugar and tells the body to store vs. burn.

So as we get older, maintaining our weight is certainly harder. However, it does not have to be a fight. Actually, most people eat less as they age. But unfortunately, to compensate for moving less at their desk jobs, their activity levels generally decreases more than their energy intakes. And with less activity than food, fat gain is evitable.

My friends and patients are teasing me because my book is called, *No Gym Go Slim*, and then talk about exercise if you want to. Yes, it is like having a book called, *Learn to Play the Guitar without the Guitar*, then me telling you to get a guitar. I will maximize your efforts IF YOU CHOOSE to exercise. So instead of exercising 30, 45, or 60 minutes, I will get you results in 20 minutes or less. But, you do not have to if you choose, and if your nutrition is optimal.

Decreasing activity levels cause the problem I discussed before, muscle loss. Muscle is a very metabolically active tissue and age-related muscle loss will cripple your metabolism. The average person experiences a 20% to 25% reduction in their 24-hour metabolism. This adds up to a drop of more than 500 calories that were currently burned at rest. Remember, 3,500 calories equals one pound. Storing an extra 3,500 calories is one pound gained. It is not hard to understand why people are gaining weight. Try removing 500 calories off your diet every day to compensate for the metabolism drop. When it comes to your body -- use it or lose it. You can, of course, reverse this process. It simply takes time.

So, if you want that youthful metabolism that your young kids have, you should build muscle. If you were to gain 5 to 10 pounds of lean muscle mass, you will burn an additional 100 to 200 calories per day at rest.

If you choose to do any type of cardio training, you should do interval training. It is highly more intense and will produce a growth hormone release which allows for less fat and a leaner body. To then accelerate the process even further, you should also weight train. I would not add weight training until you control your food. <u>You will control food or food will control you.</u> Simple weight training, along with an improved diet and proper supplementation, can increase your body's daily caloric burn up to 50%. That is enough of a boost for you to see a 10-15 pound drop in body fat during eight weeks.

When you apply as much as you can from this book, you will simultaneously improve your health, speed your metabolism, gain muscle, and shed fat. You will also start to lower your cholesterol, blood pressure, blood sugar, and other health markers. Not only can you look better, you could live longer. Just because you may be young and have not seen the effects of time – that is great -- but that does not mean it will not get you. Health comes from the inside.

I tell all my patients that spinal degeneration and spinal stenosis are inevitable. It will affect all of us. There is nothing you can do to stop it. However, you can greatly reduce the effects and help yourself by going to a Chiropractor. Just like I said before, use it or lose it. You absolutely should have a Chiropractor in your life.

As a side note, when you look at grandma and grandpa and they tell you they used to be two to three inches taller and they are shrinking, do you think that is something that just happens? There is no active blood supply to the discs within the spine of the adult. The discs are the cushions between the vertebrae that allow us to move, bend and twist. When you go to a Chiropractor, the specific spinal adjustment helps feed the discs. It provides nutrition into the discs. Most people that have disc problems simply have too much pressure and fail to hydrate the discs with Chiropractic care, decompression therapy, or anything that will provide specific spinal motion. Again, "use it or lose it".

This is why I have always encouraged people and patients to get regular Chiropractic care. Not just for pain relief, but for health prevention. I go every week and get adjusted by MY Chiropractor. <u>I cannot adjust myself.</u> A twisting of the neck or back, and hearing a "pop" is not an adjustment. If you are truly concerned about weight loss and, of course, ultimately your overall health, I suggest you add a Chiropractor to your life.

About the thyroid gland. People that have an increased activity of a thyroid gland may have more energy and lose weight. The opposite may be true, that people who suffer from a low functioning thyroid, may have weight gain and less energy. Now, in the absence of disease, I can tell you that studies I have read, and anecdotal evidence in my practice, show that people receiving Chiropractic adjustments around the lower neck/ upper back, appear to stimulate the thyroid gland, and thus are more active. These specific adjustments actually improve sleep and increase energy.

The reason most people are sluggish in the morning is the fact they skip breakfast. This is the worst thing that you can do for your health and weight management. Unless you are doing a cleanse or some type of short-term controlled fast, <u>breakfast is required</u>.

Why do people skip breakfast? We do not wake up early enough. People wake up too close to the time they have to leave. This leaves little time to prepare, eat and digest a healthy meal before they leave for work or school. What also happens is the fact they wake up late and say that they are just not hungry. This is why people need to wake up 30 to 45 minutes earlier, and take their time eating breakfast.

What if you do eat breakfast? Is it healthy? For most people, it is a poor breakfast choice and it is eaten too fast. They are usually missing protein and it is highly processed. This causes an insulin spike. Sending your kids to school by starting their day with a bowl of Apple Jacks or Fruit Loops is a <u>terrible</u> idea. In addition to having a poor choice in the morning, we usually do not eat enough in the morning.

The nutritional rule should be: eat like a king for breakfast, a queen for lunch, and a pauper for dinner. When I talked about fad diets, this is how the reverse diet was. Essentially you have your dinner for breakfast and your breakfast for dinner. This actually showed some promise, based on the fact that we usually skip breakfast, or have a small breakfast, and too much dinner.

Another problem for metabolism and weight gain is we do not consume <u>quality</u> snacks throughout our day. If you do snack, it is usually some processed carb with sugar.

Most people grab a protein bar, which, many of them, are candy bars disguised as a protein bar.

If a person that has a bad breakfast, does not snack, or has a poor snack, what happens right around lunchtime? Their blood sugar is whacked and, therefore, a search for something fast begins. It is usually a burger, fries, and a soft drink. Then, after lunch the cycle continues.

Let us say you have dinner at 7pm, which is a little late. But, you have dinner at 7pm and wake up the next day, get ready for work, and start by 9am. In that scenario, you have gone 14 hours without any type of food and, therefore, your body is already in starvation mode. Then, the bulk of total dietary energy is distributed later in the day. What this means is that hourly energy balance is hugely negative in the morning and positive in the evening. This means you should have a better distribution of food throughout the entire day, not just load up on a big dinner.

Here are 10 rules of good nutrition. This will reiterate what I have been talking about in this entire book. These rules will also help with the constant balance of your body's systems, your cravings, improvement of your metabolism, and will improve your overall health:

1. Eat every two to three hours when you can. You should eat a minimum of three meals per day. You can do fine with 3 meals spread out through the day. If you can eat and snack more frequently, that is fantastic. I know many of you are saying this is impossible. I will not be able to do it at my job. I said the same thing. I forced myself to make the change and it is now my routine. When I deviate from that routine, I feel sluggish and lethargic. I eat at approximately 7:30, 10:30, 1:30, 4:30, 6:00, and 7:30.
2. Eat protein at every meal. Nothing more to say, but you need to have protein in every meal to prevent muscle wasting.
3. Eat vegetables with every meal. The more raw the better, they have active enzymes and they will neutralize acidity.
4. Have carbs when you earn them. If you want to have a slice of pizza, I say earn it. You earn it by exercising

a specific way before you consume them. This does not mean you can eat whatever you want as long as you exercise. That is wrong. It means you can assist your body to not have as fast of an insulin response. Try interval training the day of a planned pizza night. Also, never stuff yourself or eat too fast.

5. Learn to love healthy fats. You should eat things like mixed nuts, flax seeds, and olive oil. You should love flaxseed oil and fish oil. Take them as a supplement or as a liquid that you can use on your foods. Fish oil has in it properties called Omega 3 fatty acids. It is an <u>essential</u> fatty acid. The word essential means that you need to get it in your diet. If we feed our body correctly, our body can make the chemicals it needs. Our body can make painkillers, muscle relaxers, and anti-inflammatories naturally, if we feed it the necessary components to create them. You must increase your good fats in your diet if you want to burn fat. At the end of this book I will have a list of all supplements that I recommend and personally use. I have studied Omega 3 fatty acids in detail. I would say this is very important to your overall health.

6. Forget all drinks that are not called water --fruit juice, soda, diet soda, Gatorade, energy drinks, coffee, alcohol, etc. Nothing is allowed except for water. I will, however, say that green tea is ok.

7. Focus on whole foods. Most of your dietary intake should come from whole foods. There are times when we can supplement with protein shakes, but most of the time you do best with whole unprocessed foods.

8. Have 10% fun foods. Remember what I have said, "it's not what you do all the time, it's what you do most the time that matters". One hundred percent discipline is never required to have optimal progress. Stop kidding ourselves right now, you and I are not going to have 100% compliance. I told you my original work out. Monday, I do chest and back. Wednesday, it is arms and shoulders. Friday is beer and wings. The difference between doing something most the time and all the time, believe it or not, is not that significant. For example, if you are

eating six meals a day, seven days a week, that equals 42 meals. If 10% of those were fun foods that you reward yourself with, that equals four each week. There is nothing wrong with that. The other main rule is never have a bad meal back to back. Do not have fast food for lunch, and then do it again for dinner.

9. Make sure you have food preparation strategies. You will learn later in my book under the plan, I have a system that I call 2-1-2. My 2-1-2 system is a phenomenal way to lose weight. The hardest part about eating well is making sure you follow the rules consistently. This requires planning. If you fail to plan, then you are planning to fail. On Sundays we prepare for all the meals for the week. It does not mean we cook everything on Sunday for the entire week, but we make sure we have what we need for the week.

10. Balance your food choices with variety. When you are busy during the week, you are not going to spend a lot of time preparing gourmet meals. During these times, you are going to need a set of tasty, easy to make foods that you can eat. A few times a week you should eat something different to starve off boredom.

As I said, this book is about the basics. It is like running a marathon. I have completed five. You do not start off and just run a marathon. First, you have to run. Then you have to run a lot more. But it is a progression for you to get to the end result. Once you train to be able to complete a marathon, then you add more advanced techniques to better your time and results. I am trying to get you to start by making some small changes which can lead to bigger changes that will produce results. Remember this formula, T-F-A-R. It means thoughts=Feelings=Actions=Results. Your THOUGHTS dictate how you feel. When you FEEL a certain way, you will ACT a certain way, which will produce your RESULTS. I have been using that formula for years. It really works.

Be proud of your accomplishments. YOU are competing with YOU. It does not matter if you have no desire to ever run a marathon. You may want to lose 20 pounds and, if you lose 10, that is a great achievement. Please do not set a goal to lose 20 pounds, when you need to lose 50. Your short-term goal can be to lose 20 pounds, and be proud of yourself. However, keep your eye on the grand prize – the 50 pounds. Trust me when I tell you can do it. This is all up to you. Shoot for the stars. If you hit the moon, you have done really well!

You know the statement, "misery loves company"? Well, most smokers take comfort with other smokers on a smoke break. Do not allow a negative influence to halt your goals. All I heard growing up was what I could NOT do. I always said "why can't I? "

Here is a great example. I am a huge Chicago Cubs fan. I was born and raised in Chicago. I have Cub blue in my veins. Many years ago, the Cubs hired a new manager named Dusty Baker (he is currently the manager of the Reds). When he came over to the Cubs, at the beginning of Spring Training he was asked about his team and their chances of winning. His answer was, "why not us?" That answer was so great, that so many people bought into it. The fans and media were like, "ok, ya, why not us?".

If you do not know Chicago Cubs history, they have not won a World Series since 1908. They have not been in the World Series since 1945. That is a long time. I thought Dusty Baker's attitude was incredible. He took the team to within five outs of going to the World Series (hold on as I dry my eyes). I really think that attitude is the most important factor in any goal that you set. Decide to lose weight, and if someone says you cannot or you will not, heck, prove them wrong! You have a power within you that you need to find.

Also, it is great to have a workout partner and someone to push you when you do not feel like going to the gym. The same holds true with nutrition. Maybe you do not feel like making all of the meals, and you rather grab a burger and fries, but having a partner can help. It also works the other way. You may have a friend that wants to cheat on the plan more than you do or does not want to do it today. Compete with yourself first, and then maybe you can use your discipline to motivate others and help them.

Let me finish this chapter by asking the following question: if I gave you $100,000 to lose 40 pounds, could you? If you answer yes, then why can't you do it without the money? The choice is really yours. Remember, it is your health and your future health. Dusty Baker had the Cubs players and fans believing in "why not us". I say to you, "why not you"? You deserve it. Follow the advice in this book to the best of your ability. That is all I ask and all you can ask of yourself.

Chapter 11

Juicing and Cleansing

Let me be very clear about this chapter. Juicing and cleansing are not fads, nor are they permanent solutions to weight loss. Juicing has its place. Cleansing has its place. Do not think that you are going to do a 9-day or 30-day cleanse or juicing and have permanent fat loss. It does not work that way.

I will mention the products that I personally use and professionally prescribe for my patients. You can decide to use them or not. Detoxifying with a cleanse is a great way to promote long-term health and avoid sickness and disease. So, it definitely has its place. You can do a colon cleanse and/or a heavy metal cleanse. You can also perform a detoxification for your gallbladder and liver.

It is time to discuss juicing. Last year a friend of mine, like many of you, created a New Year's resolution to lose weight. His big plan was to juice every day and every meal. Fast-forward from day 1 to day 30, and any initial weight lost that was achieved was added back, plus some extra. Why, because he treated juicing as a fad diet or a quick solution, to a more complex problem.

Juicing is a great supplementation to your overall health plan and can be a great catalyst to help you lose weight. It is not to be replaced with a healthy diet or eating fruits and vegetables alone. I will tell you that if you are juicing with fruits only, you are probably going to gain weight. I feel juicing has a better place when utilized with vegetables and some fruit.

Most of the time the skin on or inside a fruit or vegetable is its fiber. The skin, or fiber, is the sugar-neutralizing agent. If you have an apple or an orange and eat it, you will have the health benefit without the insulin release, based on the sugar – typically.

For those of you that drink fruit juices, bad news, you are not going to lose weight. You must avoid things like apple juice, grape juice, and especially orange juice. Who does not love a glass of orange juice? The problem with orange juice is, it is loaded with sugar. It is almost like drinking a soda for breakfast.

I spent years drinking orange juice before I understood about blood sugar and insulin. Remember, insulin is a fat-storage hormone. I remember being in college and loved a glass of orange juice before bed. Wonder why I had those extra pounds on me.

So, there are three reasons why you will want to consider incorporating juicing into your health regimen. When I say juicing, I mean mainly vegetable juicing. You could add some fruits to your juicing, just not fruit juice exclusive. For the most updated health information please visit Mercola.com. Dr. Mercola is a medical doctor from Chicago and has the #1 alternative website on the Internet. I highly recommend you sign up for his free e-newsletters and you can search his website for the tremendous amount of information that he has. Here are the three reasons you should incorporate juicing:

1. Juicing will help you absorb all the nutrients from vegetables. This is important because some of us have impaired digestion as a result of years of making less than perfect food choices. This limits your body's ability to absorb all the nutrients from vegetables. Juicing will help to pre-digest them for you, so you will receive most of the nutrition, rather than it being wasted.
2. Juicing allows you to consume an optimal amount of vegetables in an efficient manner. You should consume about 1 pound of raw vegetables per 50 pounds of body weight each day. Many people cannot eat that many vegetables; however, it is easily accomplished by vegetable juicing.
3. You can also add a wider variety of vegetables in your diet. Many people eat the same vegetable in their

salads every day. This violates what is called the principle of regular food rotation, and increases your chance of developing an allergy to a certain food. But again with juicing, you can choose a wide variety of vegetables that you may not normally enjoy eating whole.

I personally do not have any recommendations for a specific type of juicer, but spend a little extra on one that will last.

Remember, vegetable juice is not a complete meal. It is important to note that vegetable juice has very little protein and virtually no fat. So, by itself, it is not really a complete food. It really should be used in addition to your regular meals and not a substitute for it. Unless you are undergoing a special fasting or detoxification program, it is not a good idea to use the vegetable juicing as a meal replacement. Ideally, it can be consumed with your meal or as a between- meal snack.

Any time that you do modify your nutrition, please listen to your body. If you stop ingesting caffeine, you should expect some withdrawal symptoms. If you start to greatly increase your vegetable intake, you are probably going to feel bloated and gassy for the first two weeks.

First of all, if you are going to begin juicing vegetables, start by juicing vegetables that you already like. If you do not like cauliflower or cucumbers, it is probably not a good idea to start throwing them in the blender. The juice you drink should taste pleasant and not make you feel nauseous. Your stomach should feel good afterwards. If it is churning, growling or letting you know it is there, you probably juiced something you should not be eating.

Here are a few simple rules and lessons with juicing. Use pesticide-free vegetables. It is wise to choose organic whenever possible. However, some vegetables are worse than others when it comes to pesticides. The following list of vegetables should almost always be purchased organically: celery, spinach, kale, collard greens, lettuce, carrots, and cucumbers.

The order listed below is only intended for those that are new to juicing to see if you have a pleasant experience with it. If you add ¼ to ½ lemon or lime to the juice, you can start experimenting with the more bitter greens early on as the lemon and lime effectively counter their bitterness. Please note it would be far better to use lemon or lime than carrots, beets, and apples, which have far more fructose then lemons or limes.

The first vegetables that you should start juicing are celery, fennel and cucumbers. Those three are not as nutrient dense as dark green vegetables. According to Dr. Mercola, once you get used to these three vegetables, you can start adding the more nutritionally valuable ones.

Now you can start adding things like red leaf lettuce, green leaf lettuce, romaine lettuce, and spinach. Next on the list will be cabbage and bok choy. According to this source, cabbage juice is one of the most healing nutrients for ulcer repair. The next step would be to add herbs to your juicing. Parsley or cilantro are good choices. Again, if you want to make your vegetable juicing taste a little bit better, and easier to consume in the beginning, add lemons and limes.

Cranberries have five times the antioxidant content of broccoli. Cranberries also are chock full of nutrients, so you should limit cranberries to about four ounces per pint.

You should consume your vegetable juicing right away or store it carefully. Juicing is a time-consuming process, so juice it and then drink it. If you want to store your juice, then put your juice in a glass jar with an airtight lid and fill it to the very top. You must try to prevent oxidation as quickly as possible. Then store in the refrigerator and use when you are ready. Typically try to drink it within the first 24 hours.

From healthiersteps.com, some things people who juice are saying is: I could think more clearly, I lost weight, I found myself full of energy, I was more consistently positive and cheerful, I woke up feeling rested, I rarely felt hungry, I had an increased heightened sense of smell and taste, my hair and nails grew faster, people commented on how much younger I looked, I had better immunity and didn't catch a cold or get sick, and juicing gave me greater control over my appetite.

Here is a recipe for a fat burner juice -- six carrots, handful of kale or other green leafy vegetables and one lemon. Wash everything and cut into small pieces so it can fit into your juicer. Put the leaves in first, the carrots and lemon will help to push the leaves through the juicer and blend it better. Drink your juice right away for maximum potency, or at least within the first 24 hours if stored properly.

Fans of juicing say juicing is better than eating whole fruits and vegetables because the body can absorb the nutrients better and it gives the digestive system a rest from working on fiber. However, the nutrients might not have the same potential because you process them. There is nothing like consuming whole fruit or vegetables. Why it is true that too much fiber can sometimes block the absorption of nutrients, but most people do not even get the recommended amount of fiber per day. Make sure that you discuss juicing with your healthcare provider before integrating juicing into your diet to avoid a potential food/drug interaction. For instance, a large-muscle food high in vitamin K, such as kale and spinach, may change how an anti-blood clotting medication works.

If you are not a big fan of fruits and vegetables this is a great way to get them into your body. You can really meet your daily recommendations in one drink. But remember do not count on juicing as your sole source of fruits and vegetables. Aim to eat three or four whole vegetables a day.

So what about cleanses and detoxification programs. Every day we are exposed to hundreds of toxins, from the food we eat, to the air we breathe, to the water we drink, and even with the items we touch. Without proper cleansing, the body may struggle to maintain good health. The body needs to cleanse itself naturally. Avoid products, such as laxatives or diuretics that can harm your body. A true detoxification/cleanse nourishes and feeds your whole body with vitamins, minerals, and antioxidants.

Cleansing supports your mental and physical performance, and improves resistance to stress and overall digestive health. Cleansing, just like juicing, can give your digestion a break. Your body requires so much energy to assimilate and digest food. A controlled fast, such as juicing or cleansing, can give your body a break and allow other resources to heal and function better.

When you constantly overload your system, you really never give your body a chance to work efficiently. Just like a motor or machine that needs to cool down, but you want to keep pushing it to maximum.

Many disease processes are cumulative in nature. Think about smoking. People typically do not die by smoking one pack of cigarettes. It takes years and years to accumulate these toxins and chemicals in the body. So by cleansing, you can protect your body from the accumulation and damage of environmental toxins and oxidative stresses. This encourages safe and effective weight loss by gently removing impurities.

I mentioned before that there are different types of cleanses. I always recommend a colon cleanse at least once a year and that you perform that one first. You can also do a heavy metal cleanse, a gallbladder, and liver cleanse. You should always do a colon cleanse first.

The first company that I want to mention is <u>Isagenix. com</u>. I love them for their natural products and great tasting whey protein. This is a wonderful company that I have used for many years. Go to their website and poke around at their different types of cleansing products. I use their products and many of my patients and family have as well. They have wonderful products. Their whey protein is natural. It does not contain any artificial sweeteners, like Splenda or NutraSweet. I have one of their protein shakes every day.

The other company that I recommend for doing a heavy metal detoxification and cleansing is called <u>Jonbarron.org</u>. He is a very smart individual, who really understands how the body functions, and how to make it function better. Cleansing and supplementation is required for optimal health and for optimal health potential.

Imagine if you only had one car for your entire life. How well would you take care of it? Have you ever wondered why you change the oil in your car? Your car uses and burns oil to help with the working parts. Eventually the oil gets old and creates sludge within the engine. You get an oil change to keep your car parts sliding and gliding how they should. Just like how a Chiropractic adjustment does for your spine.

If you plan on doing maintenance to your car or go to the dentist for a cleaning, is it really that difficult to provide your body with a little <u>internal</u> maintenance too? Look, I realize that most people want to lose weight because they want to look better first and feel better second. Most people do not jump into a diet or join a gym because they are thinking 20 years in the future.

With all the knowledge and information that I have and that I am trying to share with you, I still have my last 10 pounds battle with my body. I am in the trenches with you. I understand the frustrations and disappointments, but I keep moving forward.

I am going to use a quote from the late Jimmy Valvano -- Jimmy V. This great college basketball coach gave one of the most memorable speeches when he did not have much time left. I remember him almost not having the energy to walk off stage after he gave his speech. Please Google his name and watch his speech. His line is the following, "Don't give up, don't ever give up!"

Chiropractors are the best doctors in the world for wellness. It is so easy to get people out of pain. However, it is <u>keeping</u> them out of pain that we also try to accomplish. In fact, that is also pretty easy. The hard part is keeping people in compliance.

I know many people may not want to change their habits and do what I am teaching in this book. Understand that I am trying to teach you a little bit of how the body functions and how to fix it. I know it would be very easy for me to write a book and say, day one eat this, day two eat this, etc. The problem with doing that, is that it would get boring very quickly. With no variety or knowing what you are willing to eat, the program would really be a fad.

My book is part education as I am laying down the foundation. The second part is, hopefully, motivation with some real-world examples. The third part is really up to you. Just getting you to try and make that effort.

I promise you that if you follow what I am telling you in this book, you can lose weight. This is not one of those, "I tried this and it didn't work for me". This is how your body works – period. Your body was not meant to start the day with Red Bull or Diet Coke.

If you give yourself just two to three weeks, that should be enough time to regulate your blood sugar and prime your body to start burning mainly fat versus primarily sugar. As a side note, sugar is one of the most addicting substances on the planet. It took me two weeks to get off soda completely. This is coming from a guy that is super disciplined. You can do this. You are competing with you and only you.

Juicing or cleansing is the right way to jumpstart your healthy new habits. It can give you an opportunity to actually become healthier. Just remember, juicing and cleansing is part of the healthy puzzle. I have taken my colon cleanse further and have a yearly hydrocolonic.

I love to read and research. In fact, last week I got to the end of the Internet (LOL!). The internet has so much good information, but it also has a lot of bad information. There is a tremendous amount of research that shows there is a large amount of immunity in our gut (or intestinal tract). A lot of health-related processes start in our intestinal tract. Maintaining and keeping it healthy is a great way to stay healthy. I also highly recommend a quality probiotic. A probiotic is the good bacteria. If you have ever used an antibiotic, you need to replace the good bacteria. Many people will simply eat yogurt. I do not like too much dairy in the body.

Do not go cheap on a probiotic. Recent research has suggested that cheaper probiotics are deficient in certain areas that will actually cause symptoms versus preventing them. I will have a list of companies that I recommend and use at the end of the book.

As a side note about dairy, if you can walk and talk, you do not need to drink milk. Cow's milk is great if you are a calf. Too much milk and dairy can clog your intestines and further block anything good that you are trying to put in your body. So it is just best to avoid dairy. If you choose yogurt, make it Greek yogurt, it has less sugar. The rest mostly uses artificial sweeteners – and you do NOT want that.

To summarize this chapter: juicing and cleansing are great tools for your overall health. They can be used in conjunction with a healthy lifestyle. Do not use them expecting to lose weight and keep it off. Slow and steady wins the race.

It is your health and your future health. Be there healthy!

Chapter 12

Fish Oil and Water

In this chapter I am going to further discuss a popular supplement called fish oil. Except do not look at fish oil as a supplement. It is essential to your nutrition and is required for weight loss. I will also discuss everyone's favorite equation -- H_2O.

I have decided to group these two together despite the fact that I can write an entire book on both topics. The reason to group them together is that they are both essential for life. We are talking about science, not science fiction. Both fish oil, which I mean specifically omega-3 fatty acids, and water are necessities for life, optimal function, and health.

Omega-3 fatty acids are essential fatty acids. The word essential clearly means something that is needed or is required. Fish oil will help you lose body fat for a number of reasons. Fish oil provides essential fats that the body needs. Your body cannot produce it, therefore, they must be consumed for optimal function.

Fish oil will not turn into fat in the body. The body will favorably use the fat from fish oil to build the outside lipid layer that protects our cells. Lipid means fats. Any kind of fat can be used to do this, omega 3 fats, omega 6 fats, or even trans-fats. Your cells will function their best and your metabolism will be optimal, if fish oil makes up a cell lipid layer because it binds better with insulin. The binding essentially makes the carbs be used as energy vs. stored. If it does not bind, cortisol, the stress hormone, elevates and this creates more inflammation. The result is that you get fat.

This allows for better insulin sensitivity, which is a primary factor in fat loss as I have discussed previously. If you have poor insulin sensitivity, you will have a difficult time losing fat.

The other benefit of fish oil is that it is an anti-inflammatory. I routinely recommend that all of my patients take fish oil for its anti-inflammatory properties. Another added benefit is that it is good for the heart. Most heart attacks are based on too much inflammation vs. clogged arteries. In fact, most heart attacks occur four to six hours after a very high calorie meal.

According to a study, fat loss was proven as soon as six weeks with the addition of fish oil. Healthy people were given four grams of fish oil per day and without exercise, these participants lost body fat and increased muscle mass. Again, this was done without exercise, as in *No Gym Go Slim*. Also, in this study, the participants had a decrease in their levels of cortisol after taking the fish oil. Cortisol is considered a catabolic hormone that breaks down muscle, leads to fat gain, and makes you feel stressed out.

Fish oil can actually help you build muscle because it is anabolic. Another study that was performed showed that aging rats that were given fish oil for eight weeks significantly increased protein synthesis as well as muscle. Using another study with the dosage of four grams of fish oil per day, people increased their protein synthesis and had a significant muscle building effect.

With these studies, metabolic pathways that produce muscle growth was enhanced by 30%, as was muscle cell membrane signaling. That is the same mechanism in which insulin health is improved, and further enhances muscle building. Muscle mass also increased by two percent in a short period of time.

Fish oil will enhance body composition. Inflammation in the body is horrible for health, but it will also significantly impact your ability to lose body fat and build muscle. The importance of decreasing inflammation is paramount if you want to be lean.

This information seems to really have no meaning for the general population. However, this is something essential for your health. I know it is not Pepsi, Diet Coke, or Doritos, but chronic inflammation that equals disease, sickness, illness, delayed recovery from injuries, and obesity. Your fat tissue actually produces inflammation on its own, which progressively will increase your total inflammation.

Fish oil's anti-inflammatory properties are the main reason it helps you lose fat. It can reduce and prevent chronic inflammation. It also decreases acute inflammation. After an acute (new) injury, people should be on fish oil to reduce the inflammation. If you do choose to exercise routinely, fish oil can help your recovery time as well. Fish oil helps deal with waste products produced in response to energy metabolism during exercising, thus enhancing the anabolic properties in muscle tissue.

When you get the optimal percentage of your dietary fat from fish oil, you will see the following: speedy detoxification of the stuff you do not want in your body, improved cellular health and the building of muscle, decreased hormones that cause inflammation and help you be lean and healthier, burned fat, and created muscle synthesis.

It's role in muscle building is the reason it is called an anabolic hormone. The good news is, that by taking fish oil while simultaneously limiting your carb intake, your insulin will improve the muscle building process. This helps to load nutrients into the muscle, like creatine and carnitine, which are essential for physical performance and fat burning.

An example of the effect of fish oil on insulin sensitivity is seen with the recent study of women with type II diabetes who took 2.5 grams of fish oil per day. After 30 days, the women significantly decreased body fat and shrunk their waistlines, while having significantly improved insulin sensitivity. Most of the studies that I am sharing with you suggest small doses of 4 grams per day. When I tell my patients about taking fish oil they start by taking just one pill a day. One pill is usually 1500 mg or 1.5 grams. Typically, after two or three weeks, they say it did not work or that they never experienced and changes, so they quit. Very similar to a Chiropractic patient that comes in for a few visits, says it did not work, and then quits.

In comparison, medications are designed to work really fast. Supplements, on the other hand, are the raw materials that are required for building. When it comes to supplementation, you must give the body time.

In all my years as a Chiropractor, the most difficult message to convey to a patient is, would you please stick with the plan. One hundred percent of my patients who followed my recommendations got better -- not 20%, not 50%, not 90% -- 100% got better when they followed my recommendations. You have to understand that if you have mismanaged your health and nutrition it can be reversed, but you must allow the process to occur. Be patient!

There are many times that people come to me with disc problems of the neck or the lower back. Those could take three months of dedication to fix it. Many people want a quick fix and they opt for medications or surgery to only see the problems or symptoms return and are worse. So, I am telling you, with all my heart, just give it some time.

There is some new research that suggests you can take 1 to 1.5 grams of fish oil per percentage of your body fat per day. This means, if you have 20% body fat, you could take between 20 grams and 30 grams of fish oil each day. This could help with the more rapid weight loss. When it comes to medications or supplementation, I do not ever recommend jumping in with a high dose. Start small and build and see how your body reacts.

For example, vitamin C is one of the most incredible substances that you could put in your body. Many studies say that vitamin C does not shorten the duration of a cold or it does not help the immune system. I will tell you that these studies are typically done using synthetic vitamin C, and also a dose that is not high enough. I am a huge fan of taking vitamin C. There are studies that I have read that are 20 and 30 years old, of people with serious health problems and difficulty with healing, and they took large intravenous doses of vitamin C, with incredible turnarounds with their health.

A great explanation from Dr. Andrew Weil, M.D., at drweil.com, is in the following five paragraphs:

"Omega-3 and omega-6 are types of essential fatty acids - meaning we cannot make them on our own and have to obtain them from our diet. Both are polyunsaturated fatty acids that differ from each other in their chemical structure. In modern diets, there are few sources of omega-3 fatty acids, mainly the fat of cold water fish such as salmon, sardines, herring, mackerel, black cod, and bluefish. There are two critical omega-3 fatty acids, (eicosapentaenoic acid, called EPA and docosahexaenoic or DHA), that the body needs. Vegetarian sources, such as walnuts and flaxseeds contain a precursor omega-3 (alpha-linolenic acid called ALA) that the body must convert to EPA and DHA. EPA and DHA are the building blocks for hormones that control immune function, blood clotting, and cell growth, as well as components of cell membranes.

By contrast, sources of omega-6 fatty acids are numerous in modern diets. They are found in seeds and nuts, and the oils extracted from them. Refined vegetable oils, such as soy oil, are used in most of the snack foods, cookies, crackers, and sweets in the American diet, as well as in fast food. Soybean oil alone is now so ubiquitous in fast foods and processed foods, that an astounding 20% of the calories in the American diet are estimated to come from this single source.

The body also constructs hormones from omega 6 fatty acids. In general, hormones derived from the two classes of essential fatty acids have opposite effects. Those from omega-6 fatty acids tend to increase inflammation (an important component of the immune response), blood clotting, and cell proliferation, while those from omega-3 fatty acids decrease those functions. Both families of hormones must be in balance to maintain optimum health.

Many nutrition experts believe that before we relied so heavily on processed foods, humans consumed omega-3 and omega-6 fatty acids in roughly equal amounts. But to our great detriment, most North Americans and Europeans now get far too much of the omega-6s and not enough of the omega-3s. This dietary imbalance may explain the rise of such diseases as asthma, coronary heart disease, many forms of cancer, autoimmunity and neuro-degenerative diseases, all of which are believed to stem from inflammation in the body. The imbalance between omega-3 and omega-6 fatty acids may also contribute to obesity, depression, dyslexia, hyperactivity, and even a tendency toward violence. Bringing the fats into proper proportion may actually relieve those conditions, according to Joseph Hibbeln, M.D., a psychiatrist at the National Institutes of Health, and perhaps the world's leading authority on the relationship between fat consumption and mental health. At the 2006 Nutrition and Health Conference sponsored by the University of Arizona's College of Medicine and Columbia University's College of Physicians and Surgeons, Dr. Hibbeln cited a study showing that violence in a British prison dropped by 37 percent after omega-3 oils and vitamins were added to the prisoners' diets.

In general, however, you can cut down on omega-6 levels by reducing consumption of processed and fast foods and polyunsaturated vegetable oils (corn, sunflower, safflower, soy, and cottonseed, for example). At home, use extra virgin olive oil for cooking and in salad dressings. Eat more oily fish or take fish oil supplements, walnuts, flax seeds, and omega-3 fortified eggs. Your body and mind will thank you."

You can Google a complete list of sources of omega 3s. In the United States and most other industrialized countries, diets are very high in omega 6s due to the overuse of vegetable oils. You want a balance between the 6s and the 3s, while avoiding the vegetable oils completely. The reason is these oils, many of which we cook in, or restaurants cook in, cause inflammation when you consume too much of them.

We are talking about the human body that uses all it can for survival. The estimated ratio of the diet in this country is a ratio about 16 to 1, when it should be a 2:1 or 1:1

Here is another study from ncbi.nlm.nih.gov/pubmed:

"Several sources of information suggest that human beings evolved on a diet with a ratio of omega-6 to omega-3 essential fatty acids (EFA) of approximately 1, whereas in Western diets the ratio is 15/1 to 16.7/1. Western diets are deficient in omega-3 fatty acids, and have excessive amounts of omega-6 fatty acids compared with the diet on which human beings evolved and their genetic patterns were established. Excessive amounts of omega-6 polyunsaturated fatty acids (PUFA) and a very high omega-6/omega-3 ratio, as is found in today's Western diets, promote the pathogenesis of many diseases, including cardiovascular disease, cancer, and inflammatory and autoimmune diseases, whereas increased levels of omega-3 PUFA (a low omega-6/omega-3 ratio) exert suppressive effects. In the secondary prevention of cardiovascular disease, a ratio of 4/1 was associated with a 70% decrease in total mortality. A ratio of 2.5/1 reduced rectal cell proliferation in patients with colorectal cancer, whereas a ratio of 4/1 with the same amount of omega-3 PUFA had no effect. The lower omega-6/omega-3 ratio in women with breast cancer was associated with decreased risk. A ratio of 2-3/1 suppressed inflammation in patients with rheumatoid arthritis, and a ratio of 5/1 had a beneficial effect on patients with asthma, whereas a ratio of 10/1 had adverse consequences. These studies indicate that the optimal ratio may vary with the disease under consideration. This is consistent with the fact that chronic diseases are multigenic and multifactorial. Therefore, it is quite possible that the therapeutic dose of omega-3 fatty acids will depend on the degree of severity of disease resulting from the genetic predisposition. A lower ratio of omega-6/omega-3 fatty acids is more desirable in reducing the risk of many of the chronic diseases of high prevalence in Western societies, as well as in the developing countries, that are being exported to the rest of the world."

Myself, as a Chiropractor, am all about the entire person, and not just neck pain, back pain, headaches, or weight loss, but your overall health. When our body becomes too toxic, that is when disease can set in. Most people in this country are suffering from chronic pain. Certainly, many may have an injury that may be limiting what can be done. The majority of people with chronic pain have no idea that, with proper nutrition and balancing out the internal chemistry, they can actually live a much better life and with less pain.

All my patients find it hard to believe that they could take fish oil instead of cholesterol drugs, depression meds, or even ibuprofen.

So many of my patients come in and are taking a medication for depression. It is amazing that, with a proper diet, fish oil, and exercise, how much you can truly benefit yourself. Please do not look at fish oil as a fad supplement and try it for a few weeks and then say well it did not work, you must give it time to build up in your system.

Supplements are just that, they help you close the gap of what is needed in your diet. Supplements are also not medications. Medications are designed to work really quickly, just like painkillers. You do not want to go to your doctor, get a painkiller, and find out it takes 30 days. A supplement is different, it must be given the time to work. A supplement is the raw materials that your body will convert and use for your body. In my opinion, when it comes to your health, there are no shortcuts. Invest in your health and your body, and your body will thank you for it.

I find it interesting that people will often tell me that they cannot afford my care, yet these are the same people that I bump into at the local hardware store spending money on paint, wallpaper, new kitchen cabinets, fertilizer, grass seed, etc. to make their house pretty. And heaven forbid I bump into them at Wal-Mart or the grocery store and see what is in their carts.

There is certainly nothing wrong with doing these things. Sometimes you have to prioritize. It is okay to have fun. It is even fine to have fun food and party. You, at times, must make sacrifices and choices that will benefit your health. Certainly a new car and a beautiful lawn are nice things. But, if you cannot enjoy them, what is the point? Please, when it comes to your health, invest in it too!!

Now, I am switching over to water. I mentioned that I could write an entire book on the importance of drinking water. The majority makeup of your body is water. The majority makeup of this planet is water. Just like an essential fatty acid, water is a necessity for life.

Guess what else I tell my patients, you must drink water. Several patients have said to me, "I just don't like water". To me, that is like saying "I don't like breathing air". There are so many products that you could mix or add to your water to make your water taste "better" – don't, just drink pure water!

Most of you will start today with a cup of coffee, sodas, diet sodas, or energy drinks – STOP! If you are trying to be healthy, and you want to accomplish weight loss, then you can only drink water. Beer, wine, soda, diet soda, fruit juices, and energy drinks are out.

I am originally from Chicago. I now live in North Carolina. It is a little different culture between the two places. In my practice, it seems all of my patients drink this soda called Sun Drop. Maybe it is all over the country, but I have never heard of it until I came to North Carolina. But man, do these southerners love their Sun Drop.

I mentioned diet soda is worse than regular soda. Soda's main ingredient is phosphoric acid. Phosphoric acid messes with the calcium/magnesium ratios in the body, and actually lowers your satiety level of fullness and makes you eat more. I just saw a disgusting commercial made by the Coca-Cola Company. Wow, what a bunch of lies! Basically, what the commercial said is that a calorie is a calorie, and it does not matter where it comes from. So I guess 500 calories of Coca-Cola or Diet Coke are the same as 500 calories of vegetables – um, I don't think so. According to the commercial, consume too many calories and you will gain weight. You could enjoy Coca-Cola as long as you exercise and restrict calories.

I am sorry that I got off topic, but these big corporations do not care about people, they care about profits. This, I am sad to say, also includes the drug companies. This is not a book to bash big corporate America and the drug industry. But let the record show that they have made billions of dollars by destroying the health of people. It is a choice to drink and consume their products. If people did not buy their products they could not sell them.

When you want to become healthier and lose weight, then stick to water. Water provides several functions within the body. Since your body is made up of water, it is a good idea to make sure that you have enough of a supply of water. Your cells use water. Water lubricates your joints. Your knees, shoulders, elbows, hips, and spine all need regular water intake. Water is also used as a way to transport waste from your body.

I love this example, it is gross, but I think you will get the point. Your typical toilet tank holds seven gallons of water. When you go to the bathroom and flush the toilet, seven gallons of water rinses and cleans the bowl. Now try this, use the bathroom, flush, and only one gallon of water is released, how clean will it get? The answer is not very. Think about that when you are lacking your water intake. You are not flushing your body properly. Beverages (like coffee, sodas, juices, etc.) do not equal water – <u>drink water!</u>

Water is your body's most important nutrient, it is involved in every bodily function, and makes up 70 to 75% of your total body weight. Water helps you to maintain body temperature, metabolize body fat, aid in digestion, lubricates and cushions organs, transports nutrients, and flushes toxins from your body. Oh did I mention, <u>metabolizes body fat</u>.

OK, so how much water? Every answer seems to be the same, 64 ounces -- remember to consume 8, 8 ounce glasses a day. But, how can everyone be required to have the same amount? Someone who is five feet tall and weighs 95 pounds should consume the same amount of water with someone who is six feet tall and 200 pounds? Answer -- no.

The first thing you should do is, cut your body weight in half, and that is how many ounces of water you should work up to in a day. Example, a 100-pound person should drink 50 ounces of water per day maximum. A 200-pound person should consume 100 ounces of water per day maximum. If you are not a regular water drinker, you will spend a lot of time going to the bathroom in the beginning. I think starting at 25% and reaching 35% would be great. You will be getting water from some of the foods you eat as well. So start with 25% and move slowly to 35%.

If you are not getting enough water, your body will react by pulling it from other places including your bloodstream. This can cause the closing of some of your smaller blood vessels and make your blood thicker, more susceptible to clotting and harder to pump through your system such as your heart. This can have serious implications in high blood pressure. More studies have linked the lack of water to headaches, arthritis, and even heartburn.

Some people are just too bloated to even drink water. You need to really look at your diet and also salt intake. Consuming too much salt or salty food will signal the body to retain fluids. Your body will tolerate a certain amount of salt, however, the more salt you consume, and the more fluids you need to dilute it. To overcome that, drink plenty of water.

Being dehydrated (not having enough water in you) promotes the increase of body fat. Water contributes to energy storage along with collection. Without water, extra amounts of glucose remain in the bloodstream until it reaches the liver. This extra glucose is stored as fat. Your body takes water from inside cells in an effort to compensate for a dehydrated state. This includes fat cells. Less water in your fat cells means less mobilization of fat for energy. Conclusion is fat storage.

One of the liver's primary functions is to metabolize stored fat into energy. The kidneys are responsible for filtering toxins and waste out of the bloodstream. If you are dehydrated, the kidneys cannot function properly and the liver must overwork to compensate. The result is that it burns less fat. So, if you are trying to decrease the amount of your body fat, and, therefore, lose weight, drink plenty of water.

I am trying to point out, and hopefully you now see that, your health suffers by not giving it what it needs, like proteins, water, fish oil, etc. <u>When your body is not given the fuel it needs, it will suffer.</u>

Here is this example again: if you want to cut the price of gas for your car on your next fill up, it is simple. Fill up half your tank with gas, then come home and fill the rest with water from your garden hose. You got a full tank at half the price. Seriously, you would <u>never</u> do that to your car, <u>but you do it every day to your body.</u>

Here is another great thing about water. It is always better to drink pure water instead of anything else. Other beverages can actually increase your need for water because most of them contain caffeine. <u>Caffeine is a diuretic and this removes water and other essential nutrients from your body.</u>

We can talk about sources of water. You can go out to the store and buy cases of bottled water. But, I do not recommend bottled water, when you can easily by a filter or filtering system for your home. Bottled water is okay if you are going on a trip to take with you on vacation. The problem I have with bottled water is the fact that the water has been sitting in those plastic bottles for who knows how long. The chemicals used in plastic bottles, specifically BPA and whatever else, is not healthy. I store water in a glass container or a BPA free bottle, and I also drink from glassware. Note, many chemicals in plastic containers mimic estrogen and can cause an imbalance with men and women.

Remember, if you start to exercise or regularly exercise, you actually need <u>more</u> water. A reduction of water in the body, as little as five percent, can result in 20 to 30% slow down in your body's performance. If you lose 10% of the water content, your body will get sick. Around 20% and you could actually die.

Also, keep an eye on the color of your urine. If your urine is light yellow, you might be getting rid of excess water. When it is darker, like a dark yellow, your body is probably holding onto water, which is a good indication to start drinking more water.

If you do not drink enough, the body will retain water as a reserve. The same thing occurs with fish oil. Provided you do not take in enough fatty acids, your body will hold onto fat as a defense mechanism.

In my office I have a wonderful chart I copied from the Mayo Clinic's website, and it says the following:

Functions of Water in the Body:

- Regulates body temperature.
- Lubricates joints.
- Moistens tissues such as those in the mouth, eyes and nose.
- Protects body organs and tissues.
- Helps prevent constipation.
- Aids in digestion.
- Lessens the burden on the kidneys and liver by flushing out waste products.
- Helps dissolve minerals and other nutrients to make them accessible to the body and carries nutrients and oxygen to the cells.

If that is not enough to convince you to drink plenty of water, then you are in the wrong book. Drop this book right now and go get one about vampires and have fun.

Three things you can do to improve the taste of water is add a lemon, a lime, or some cucumber slices in your water. Drinking cold water will actually allow your body to burn extra calories. Why? Energy is required to raise the temperature of cold water.

Remember were not just talking about weight loss, weight loss is easy. If you just want to drop some pounds on the scale, try a laxative or find any high school wrestling coach, they know how to get people to "make their weight." But, if you want to be healthy and lose body fat, then start drinking water.

It is your health and future health. Here are to the future new you!

Chapter 13

Exercise and The Plan

I have made a large attempt to thoroughly cover the importance of proper nutrition as it not only applies to weight loss, but to overall good health. What about those who already work out or want to begin an exercise program? I must address this.

Yes you should exercise. You should increase your circulation while also improving your muscle tone. You should exercise in a way that benefits you and does not hurt you. You should treat exercise as an investment in not only your health, but an investment in your body. The last I checked we do not get to trade in our bodies when they are older and broken for a newer model, so take care of the one you have!

So many people need a new calendar to make health changes. Quitting smoking and weight loss are the most popular New Year's resolutions that people make. If this is the case, why do so many people fail?

People start a New Year's resolution to lose weight and fail for two main reasons. One, you go ahead and take your busy life and hectic schedule and add exercise to that schedule. This further complicates your life and, when the stress hits, the first thing you drop is usually the last thing you added. People should make health first on their list, but they do not. Number two, is that you do not see results fast enough and, therefore, get discouraged and quit. Many people that start exercise will not get results as they barely push themselves. Like walking on a treadmill or using the elliptical machine. The elliptical is the worst piece of cardio equipment there is. It takes almost no effort to use it. It is based on momentum and is very easy to perform. Yes, you can sweat on that machine, but you will never get a physique change from it, nor will you get into fat loss. This section of my book is for you to <u>maximize your return - on your fat burn!</u>

There are so many people that start an exercise program and simply do not have a solid plan. Most people that start an exercise program do not work out enough days per week and do not have a high enough intensity to create a physical change in their bodies. The bottom line is if you do not see results, you will quit. This again all comes down to nutrition. Abs are made in the kitchen, not the gym.

Every gym that I have ever belonged to has trainers that show you how to use this machine or perform that exercise, however, they offer zero nutritional guidance. In this chapter I am going to show you how you can customize your workouts while having them be more intense, fun, and with better results.

The reason (again) the title of my book is *No Gym Go Slim,* is because you must control your nutrition, or your nutrition will control you. You can do all the things in my book and it will increase the quality and quantity of your life. The side effect of doing what I am telling you to do in this book is that you will lose weight, be leaner, and also be healthier. The bottom line is to be healthier. I can get you to lose weight on the scale, but I have mentioned that is not the best choice for judging one's health improvement.

I have plenty of patients that exercise five days a week. They get up and exercise before work. Despite getting up early and making a huge commitment, many are still overweight and some are obese. Why is this? Their exercise is not intense enough and their nutrition stinks. I have a patient that not only exercises daily, but also spends money on a personal trainer. This person has not lost weight, changed her body composition, nor is she even healthy. I have known her for over two years. She is clinically obese. Why -- nutrition, nutrition, nutrition.

If you choose to add exercise, your results can be better. Understand that my plan of attack for you is to first handle the nutrition, while <u>slowly</u> adding exercise if you choose. I hope that you exercise. I want you to exercise. For the first two to three weeks, I am recommending that you have zero exercise. You can be active and go for walks, but no structured plan. After that period, you can slowly add small amounts of exercise if you choose. You do not have to. But this is something to work towards. But, I promise you, that as your health and weight improve through nutrition, you will WANT to exercise.

If you are already performing regular exercise, then by tweaking your nutrition with everything I have talked about in this book, your results will be far better. I am also going to tell you that if you tweak your exercise by adding interval training and supersets, your results will be that much greater.

In life, you want to simply maximize your return. If I was writing a book about investing your money, ask yourself the following question: if you invested $10,000, would you like a 1% return or a 10% return? Obviously of those two choices you would like the higher return. You want the most bang for your buck. Your nutrition and exercise should be no different.

The only thing that I ask of you is that YOU are competing with YOU. Do not compete with me or someone else. Challenge yourself. I am not asking that you run a marathon or compete in a triathlon. What I am asking you to do is challenge you to be a healthier version of yourself then you are right now. The human body is the greatest machine ever invented. It is capable of amazing things. By incorporating the information in this book, you are on your way to a transformation that you may not yet believe. <u>But, you must give it time</u>.

I tell patients this analogy that I mentioned in a previous chapter: imagine you are remodeling your kitchen, your kitchen will look worse before it gets better. You will not look worse, but you may feel worse initially. Your body will go through a process. There may be some withdrawal symptoms or sore muscles. As you move forward, just continue to imagine the all new you. Focus on the destination, but try to enjoy the journey.

If you have not exercised in a while, you must start slow. Do not injure yourself. Do not have a high amount of intensity where you are going to be so sore that you hate exercise. Simply start slow. Another reason why people quit exercise is that they are so sore and fatigued. They do not give their body an opportunity to push through that initial plateau or soreness. Some of the best workouts I have had was going in sore and leaving feeling great.

After the first month, your intensity should increase. The intensity of the workout is necessary to stimulate your body to produce growth hormone. Growth hormone will burn the fat and create lean muscle. Please note, that when you exercise, your post workout meal is considered an extension of the workout. <u>Do not screw it up by having a sports drink or bad meal immediately after. Sugar will stop the release of growth hormone and you have potentially wasted a good workout.</u> This is when a protein shake is your optimal choice -- immediately after a workout.

The type of cardio activity that you need to work up to is called interval training (or intervals for short). Intervals are how you played as a kid. Kids outside chase each other, catch their breath, and repeat the process. This is what I want you to do.

You can use a treadmill, a bike, or a rowing machine. After an initial warm-up of about five minutes, I would like you to go as fast as you can for 60 to 90 seconds. You then rest by slowly walking or slowly moving for 90 to 120 seconds. You then repeat that sequence 8 to 10 times. This type of training will stimulate a growth hormone release and will burn fat. Slow-boring cardio is catabolic and can actually store fat versus burning fat. The great thing about intervals is that you can get a great workout in about 25 to 30 minutes.

If you Google interval training, you may even see 20 to 30 seconds of intensity with only 10 to 20 seconds of rest. One minute on and two minutes off seems to be a nice starting point.

As I said, I have personally completed five marathons. In training for each, from start to finish, I lost a total of 3 pounds. My patients see my lean physique and say you must be running another marathon -- not at all. Slow, methodical, cardio is counter-productive. The next time you are at a health club, take a look at the people on the cardio equipment versus the people lifting weights. It is quite clear that the weightlifters for the most part are the ones that are lean, fit, and muscular. Compare marathon runners to sprinters and you can easily see which group is muscular.

When you Google interval training programs, you will find a lot of variations of what I just mentioned. You must make it intense for you. My intervals on a treadmill consist of a 60 second sprint at 9.9 mph with a 75 second break. I repeat that 10 to 12 times. It is one of the greatest workouts that I do. It is also fun, quick, and in no way boring.

Interval training does the following: it gives you a fun workout, it greatly accelerates your heart rate, stimulates growth hormone release, burns fat, and saves time.

Note: if you are not in shape or have not exercised recently, you must take it slow. Do not jump into a program that you are not ready for. You do not decide today that you are going run a marathon on Sunday. You may start with some 10Ks, then a half marathon, but you must really train for a marathon. If you choose to exercise, I ask that you build up to intervals by the fifth week of starting exercising. **Always talk to your healthcare provider before you start any exercise program.**

I would like to give you an example. There are two guys at the gym that are there at the same time that I am. Their routine has been this for about three years. They walk on a treadmill for 30 minutes. After the treadmill, they take some elastic bands and do about 5 minutes of some sort of resistance exercise. Needless to say, doing the same thing over and over again and expecting different results is the definition of insanity.

Sure, they are going to the gym and moving around while raising their body temperature a little bit, but there is no intensity with their routine. As a result of not challenging the body, these two guys have not changed their overall appearance in three years. I do not know what their nutrition is like, but I certainly know that they are not producing results. I honestly do not think with their level of exercise, that they will actually ever receive any health benefits. It is not about losing weight and looking good in a bathing suit, it is about overall health. An intense workout will burn fat and produce a growth hormone release. That is what you need.

Most people do not have a high enough intensity with their workout. This is why 90% of people that start an exercise program quit because they do not get the results they want, because they are not doing it at a high enough intensity.

I now want to discuss resistance training, also known as weight training. I want you to consider implementing a weight-training program. When it comes to weight training, I want you to apply the same philosophy as I mentioned with cardio training. That is to say that weight training should also be intense. Too many people that do weight lifting at the gym, do it in a fashion that it looks like they just want to hurry through it and get it done. They go too fast and their form is terrible.

Weight training needs to have proper form, with proper intensity. Most people feel that they need to get their cardio training to help their heart and lungs. What most people do not understand is that an intense weight training routine can offer greater cardio-vascular benefits than slow cardio.

If you are interested in starting weight training, I hope that you will consider using free weights versus machines. Adjustable dumbbells and an adjustable bench are just about all you need to get in great physical shape.

If you decide to weight train, let me mention a couple terms that you will need to know -- the difference between sets and reps (reps are short for repetitions). Reps are the number of times you perform an exercise. A set is how many groupings of that exercise you do. For example, if you are going to perform a bicep curl, you may perform 3 sets of 10. This means you will perform a total of 30 bicep curls, with a break in between every 10. For those that do weight training, you would actually be better off increasing the weight and performing 6 sets of 5 -- still having a total of 30 reps, but again with more intensity.

What I have asked you to do, if you decide to weight train, is perform what is called a superset. A superset is a group of two, three, or four exercises that you perform rapid fire. A superset will help stimulate the body to produce, guess what, a growth hormone release. Another benefit of the superset, it is not boring and you get done quicker.

You ladies, please listen up. Do not be afraid of weight training. Women do not have the same level of testosterone or muscle mass as men do. The results of you weight training will make you lean and thin. Do not worry; you will not end up looking like a professional wrestler.

So, what days do you exercise or how do you break it down? The most effective break down that I have found with myself, and my patients, is what I call the 2-1 system. This system is highly effective for <u>maximizing your return on the fat burn</u>. With this system, you exercise two days in a row and take one day off and then repeat. This is much better than doing something like Monday, Wednesday and Friday. The 2-1 system continues to challenge the body. Some weeks you will have four days of training, others you have five days.

When it comes to your particular exercises, I want you to choose your own exercises. You will decide on two groups of exercises: a group of upper body and a group of lower body. You should pick 9 to 12 exercises per group. If you Google supersets or type in "supersets" at the website <u>www.about.com</u>, you will find a complete list of exercises to choose from.

I would break the supersets into groups of three. For example, if you pick 12 exercises for the lower body, you will have four groups of three. When you are grouping the exercises, choose at least two or three that oppose each other. For example, you will group quadriceps and hamstrings together. You could group your core/abs with the lower back. Another example is biceps and triceps, or upper back with a chest workout. You could also pick six exercises, and do the program two times. I prefer more exercises as it produces less boredom.

Understand that many exercises will have an overlap. You are not just going to exercise chest because you also use arms and shoulders. Again my preference is to use free weights when possible versus machines. As long as you use a slightly heavier weight and lower reps, you will be fine.

If you can perform more than 12 repetitions without struggling, then you need to increase the weight. A minimum of six reps with a maximum of 12 is what you are shooting for.

When you perform a superset, give yourself a 30 second break, but no more than 45, between each exercise. Between each superset, you rest two minutes before beginning the next superset.

Some of this may sound confusing and you may not fully understand it, but do not worry. I will give plenty of examples and spell it out for you. In all honesty, many gyms offer a lot of fancy equipment, but the only thing you need is some dumb bells and an adjustable bench to get into amazing shape.

Exercise is important and I hope you will add it to your lifestyle, but nutrition is the key. If and when you decide to add exercise to your healthy lifestyle, make sure that every four weeks you completely mix up the exercise routine. Use different equipment with your intervals and change the exercises of weight training that you perform. Your body does get used to the same routine and it is important to continue to challenge and stimulate it for continued success. Just like the example of the two guys at the gym doing the same routine for the last three years. When I first joined the gym they may have not been in good enough shape to even do what they are doing now. Certainly, by this time, they are more than capable to perform a higher level of exercise to achieve greater results.

The program with intervals is the same 2-1 program. You will perform intervals on the same days that you perform weight training. Yes, this is an intense program of exercising two times per day. This is something you should consider building up to.

I know for many people, exercising two days on and one day off is going to be difficult, let alone doing it twice in one day. I am giving you the maximum return for your fat burn. If you had to choose between the intervals and the weight training, I am going to tell you, from experience, to stick with the weight training. By improving your muscle mass, your internal chemistry will be more efficient and your body will burn more calories at rest. With increased muscle mass, comes better overall health.

Based on discussions I have had with my patients over the years and surveys I have done, many people simply want to tone up. That is perfectly fine. With proper nutrition, as outlined in this book, you will do just that.

For simple toning of your body this is the program that I recommend: two consecutive days of weight training followed by one day of intervals. The fourth day is a rest day. Then you repeat the program. You create 9 to 12 exercises of the upper body and 9 to 12 exercises of the lower body. You will group three to four exercises in a superset, and you will perform the lower body on day one, the upper body on day two, and intervals on day three. This type of program is a really good program to start with.

Now, let me tell you a little bit about exercise and weight loss. You will become greedy. There is no doubt in my mind. Most people, when they set goals, set them way too small. They feel that they cannot achieve something bigger or just do not have the confidence enough in themselves.

When you start feeling better, you are going to start improving all areas of your life. As you lose weight, your clothes start fitting better, your friends and coworkers start complimenting you, you are going to want to continue. I have had people lose 10 pounds just from nutrition alone and turn that into 20 pounds. This is just a starting point for many of you. You have no idea where this can take you. I had a patient of mine lose 60 pounds with my advice. She has turned that into a part-time position teaching yoga and Zumba classes.

Remember the old saying, "you need to learn to walk before you can run". Please take it slow. Only compete with yourself. If it takes you 30 minutes to complete one mile, great! The next time, see if you can do it in 25 minutes. Then see if you could do 2 miles in 30 minutes. YOU compete with YOU!

This section is filled with ways to maximize your return on your fat burn. I do not want you adding any exercise for the first four weeks. Nutritional changes only! When you start eating better, your body may go through some withdrawal symptoms. I do not want to add to withdrawal symptoms of fatigue or headaches and then throw in a whole bunch of new exercise that may make you sore. <u>So please, hear me when I tell you, nutritional changes only for the first four weeks.</u>

I want you to be aware that when you begin any exercise program, <u>you will gain weight first</u>. When you exercise, you are actually fatiguing and damaging your muscles while forcing them to adapt. They must get stronger. During this initial micro-trauma to your muscles, your body will retain water. Therefore, your weight will increase initially. I do not want you going on a scale anyway, but I know you will. So I need to point that out that it is a completely normal process. After three or four weeks your body will typically let go of the extra water storage.

A few more things I want to mention about exercise. When possible, you should do your intervals in the morning or at lunchtime. For those of you that have kids, you know you do not let them play and run around before bedtime because then they get all riled up and then have difficulty sleeping. On the opposite side there is weight training, which I prefer you to in the evening either before or after dinner. I do weight training in the evening and after my muscles are very sore and fatigued, there is nothing more that I would rather do than just lay down and go to sleep.

People that exercise get better sleep. Remember that your body heals and repairs at rest, so sleep is a vital component to your weight loss and overall health. In a recent survey that was performed from <u>myhealthnewsdaily.com</u>, Rachel Rattner confirms my point of people that exercise gets better sleep.

At the end of the chapter you will see some specific examples of how I group my supersets so that you can see how to do it for yourself. I have read just about every diet book on the market. What I do not like, is the fact that, if I tell you to eat fish four days a week and you hate fish, the program will not work. If you tell me you hate running and

I tell you to run four times a week, you will not like the program and get no results.

My goal is to give you the toolbox and you decide which tools you want to fill it with. This includes both the exercise portion and the nutritional component -- nutritional being the most important. You need to choose from the strategies and incorporate them with your schedule.

Please, as you go through this book, do not start making excuses that you do not have the time to do it. There is a great newspaper cartoon that has a doctor telling a patient the following: "what fits your busy schedule better, exercising one hour a day or being dead 24 hours a day." Nutrition comes first, you can always add exercise second.

Some more reasons why I do not want to just give you a long-term plan to follow is from an article I read by Cynthia Sass at Foxnews.com. The article is "Five reasons your diet is making you fat." They are:
1. A diet can throw your body out of balance.
2. Diets do not allow for wiggle room.
3. You have to eat foods you do not like.
4. Diets are filled with fake foods.
5. Diets forbid foods you cannot give up.

What I am going to do is provide a few menus that you should do your best to follow for the first few weeks. That means two or three weeks at most. Some people need it as a jump-start to get started. They are designed specifically to regulate your blood sugar, decrease insulin sensitivity, and burn fat. Frankly, they have been around for years. I have used them to get started -- they work.

It is not something that you do for months and months like other fads. But, I will be providing them to give you a little bit of guidance for the first two to three weeks. Once you get into that fourth and fifth week, habits are going to start forming. Those will be positive reinforcements that are going to do it. You are going to feel so much better, but if you do go back to the dark side, you are going to feel worse than you did before.

When you incorporate a healthy lifestyle, exercise, and even do regular cleansing, try and go back and indulge on some really bad foods. First, you will notice your taste buds have changed and that food does not taste as good. Second, your body will tell you those choices were not a good idea. You will feel bloated, gassy, lethargic, sick, have headaches, etc. You will be so surprised on how little you desire junk food. Sugar is so addicting. As you avoid that, you will not have the cravings you once did. You are going to feel so much better, sleep better, and have much more energy. Do not be surprised that your attitude may change for the better too. There are plenty of scientific studies that back this up. Once you personally experience this transformation, you are set for life.

Specific Examples

When you decide to begin an exercise program, take it slow. If you have more experience with exercise, then you can move to a more advanced form of training. I prefer that you incorporate the nutritional changes first.

Basic Toning. This is a program example that I recommend for people that want to incorporate weight training, along with intervals, to achieve greater muscular tone and fitness.

Day 1

Superset A

Dumbbell Squats, Incline Bench Prone Rows, Incline Hyper-extension w/ Swiss ball, Flat Dumbbell Bench press.

Superset B

Dumbbell Romanian Dead lift, Standing Rope Face-pull, Planks.

Perform each exercise in Superset A, with 30 seconds rest in between. Perform 4 sets. You should perform 8 to 12 reps of each exercise. Take your time and feel the muscles working during the exercise. When completed, wait 2 minutes, and then perform Superset B. Continue the same pattern with Day 2 exercises.

Day 2

Superset A

Trap Bar Dead lift, Standing Shoulder Press, Front-foot elevated Dumbbell Squat, Lat Pull down

Superset B

Reverse Hyper-Extensions, Bent-Over Rows, Walking Dumbbell Lunges

Day 3

Perform 8 to 10 sessions of intervals. Using a rowing machine, treadmill or stationary bike. Warm up for five minutes and then complete the following:

Sprint, row, or bike as fast as you can for 1 minute with a 2 minute recover period. During the recovery period, you can walk or move slowly, but keep moving when possible. After 2 minutes, repeat this 8 to10 times.

<u>Day 4</u>

Rest

<u>Day 5</u>

Start over again with Day 1, Day 2, etc. up to 30 days completed.

The above program is the actual baseline that I start my patients at. I may alter an exercise or two, and tweak the program according to athletic ability, health condition, and access to equipment, but you get the idea.

After about four weeks, you do want to mix the exercises up. Many reasons, but the most obvious is the need to constantly challenge and stimulate your muscles and to prevent boredom.

Use the internet and the websites I have mentioned to create a program that is best for you. Challenge yourself. Try using opposing muscle groups when you get past 30 days. Like lower back and core, quads and hamstrings, and biceps and triceps.

Just like the nutrition, I do not want to give you a cookbook to follow and say here you go. I want you to choose. There are many ways to get to a destination, just try and enjoy the journey and with health you want to get there as quickly as you can, <u>but please, just give it time</u>.

Here is a program I do now that I consider more advanced:

<u>Day 1</u>

Superset A

Barbell Dead lift, Barbell Front-Foot elevated Split Squat

Superset B

Dumbbell Forward Lunge, Barbell Good Mornings
Superset C
Dumbbell Squat, Lying Leg Curl
Superset D
Planks w/ Toe Touch (feet on high bench)

Obviously, with this program, I only have two exercises per superset. I use a heavier weight and perform the weight training exercises at 5 to 7 reps. All of the exercises are lower body on this day.

Day 2
Superset A
Barbell Decline Bench Press, Barbell Bent over Rows
Superset B
Dips, Mid-grip Pull downs
Superset C
Seated Dumbbell Press, Dumbbell Pullovers
Superset D
Decline Lying Triceps Extensions, Incline Bench Curls

Again, I only have two exercises per superset. I use a heavier weight and perform the weight training exercises at 5 to 7 reps. All of the exercises are upper body on this day.

On weight training days, I also perform interval training. I use my 2-1 system of exercise -- 2 days on and 1 day off, then repeat.

My exercise routine is based on my goals and current plan. You can mix yours up to suit your needs. I simply want to show you some advanced training tips. By doing supersets with minimal rest, you can get better results, thereby stimulating a growth hormone release with intense training.

The Plan – Nutrition

At this point, you should be well versed in what to eat and what not to eat. For the first two weeks, I am going to ask that you determine your daily caloric needs. Google the Harris – Benedict Equation to get an idea of what your body requires in a day. This is an estimate, without exercise, or considering the type of lifestyle that you have. This is called your basal metabolic rate (BMR).

I want you to write everything down that you eat and drink. You should do it all the time. It is a nice way to track your progress and to see how certain foods react with you. Do you get bloated, gassy, moody, etc.?

When you begin your journey, I want you to look at calories for the first two weeks. We want to control your blood sugar and re-start our body becoming healthier. The goal is to have no more insulin spikes.

I want you to take the first two to three weeks and follow my plan. After the initial two to three weeks, you will create your own meals based on science and not fads. <u>YOU DO NOT HAVE TO COUNT CALORIES</u>. That does not work long-term because your body has an internal regulator, called homeostasis.

Remember my 2-1 plan. You are going to restrict calories on Day 1 and Day 2 BELOW your BMR number. Day 3 is at that number or even slightly above that number. Then repeat for Day 4, 5, and 6. On Day 7 I want you to have whatever you want, as long as you follow my rules. Do not eat fast, or a ton of carbs, and do not have a junk meal back to back. Just eat sensibly with a meal of something that you enjoy on Day 7 without guilt.

After two to three weeks of this, your body will be in a better position to start burning fat verses sugar. This is what we want. In a way we are re-starting your system to begin the process.

During the third week and beyond, you are going to work on the basics. This means a lot of lean protein, a lot of green vegetables, and a lot of water. I want you to remember the A, B, Cs of weight loss. These are the no-no's. No Alcohol, no Bread and no Carbs (processed).

When you do this for the initial four weeks, your body will love you for it. You will weigh less. Specifically, you will feel better, and you will be burning fat and losing weight.

If you decide to incorporate carbs, I say you need to "earn" them. By doing intense cardio, like intervals, your body can handle some of the carbs. I would not go too wild with that statement. People take that to mean, as long as they exercise, they can eat a bunch of carbs. I talked about this previously. This is incorrect. You can eat well and exercise for three days, but have one bad day of nutrition and can really set you back. That is why I say no bad meals back-to-back.

I prefer you avoid all processed carbs. But that is not realistic. I am going to ask that you plan three meals per day and two to three snack meals. Try and get protein in every meal. If you eat six times a day, seven days a week, that is 42 meals per week. To have 90% success, means you can have four fun meals each week. Just do not do them back-to-back. Ninety percent of anything is fantastic. Remember, when you shoot for the stars and only hit the moon, you are doing great!

I have seen this so many times. You will get greedy with your health. You will want more weight loss, less fat, more muscle, and more energy. You will get to the point that those fun meals really deplete your energy and attitude, and that you will want to go immediately back to healthier eating.

Here is an example of my daily nutrition:

7am   250g lean steak / small handful cashew nuts
10am   250g chicken/100g broccoli
1pm   250g salmon/100g asparagus
5pm   Protein shake (40g whey protein/ 20g glutamine)
6pm   250g chicken/ 100g cauliflower
9pm   250g Halibut/ 100g spinach

This is my advanced program as I am weight training for muscle growth and strength. You will not need as much protein. But you can clearly see that I am consuming a lot of protein to maintain my muscle mass and also to grow it.

As you move into week three and four, simply replace the 10am and 9pm meals with protein-based snacks. You can use whey protein shakes or quality protein bars. If you do not like fish, then you replace it with something that you do like. But remember to consume about two to four grams of fish oil supplements daily.

Here is an example of what your nutrition may look like.

Breakfast   250g lean steak / small handful cashew nuts
Mid morning   Whey protein shake with water or almond milk

Lunch   250g salmon/100g asparagus
Mid afternoon   Protein bar / some mixed nuts
Dinner   250g chicken/ 100g broccoli
Bedtime   Whey protein shake / fish oil supplements

I give these as examples. You can mix it up. I want you to mix it up. Variety will help with boredom and food sensitivities. For me, my brain tells me I need a carb once in a while. So in all honesty, I may once per week, have eggs for breakfast on a bagel. I do not do it all the time, but it helps me with my motivation. As my body has flipped the fat burning switch, I will still eat a sandwich or a slice of pizza. Let us be honest here, I do not do it all the time, but I am still going to enjoy my favorite foods. You will too.

I mentioned it before, but there is no magic menu to follow. I am going to give you a pre-plan program what I like to call my Quik Start recipes. It is more of a regulating of the body. Your body will release some of its "junk" and you will feel better. It will also motivate you to get going. This is something that you do for only a few days. The purpose is to start regulating your body and allowing better function. It is restrictive. That is why we only do it for a few days. After you do it, do not run out and stuff yourself. Do not use it as a quick solution or a fad. Use it as a way to jump start feeling better and regulating your internal environment.

Follow the rules in this book and you will be so happy with your results. When you begin, remember, your body takes time to adjust and adapt. Like a mortgage payment, you may not see the balance go down quickly as there is interest and principle, but over time, you are actually making a dent. Hang in there. You are on your way!

<u>QUIK Start Recipes</u>

Breakfast

Egg Muffins

In a small bowl, mix in 1 egg, 1 tbsp of diced tomatoes, zucchini, and deli turkey. Coat a muffin tin with cooking spray. Pour mixture into one muffin space. Repeat until all are full. Top each with grated cheese. Bake at 350 for

12 to 15 minutes or until brown – check with toothpick to see if done in middle. Let it cool, then put them into Ziploc bags. Store in frig or freezer. To reheat, microwave them for approximately 30 seconds.

Protein Pancakes

> 3 whole eggs
> 3 egg whites
> ½ cup rolled oats
> 2 medium zucchini
> ½ yellow onion
> 1 tsp parsley
> ½ tsp minced garlic
> 6 tsp extra-virgin olive oil
> dash of salt and ground pepper

Mix together the eggs, egg whites, and rolled oats. Chop up the zucchini and onion into a separate bowl, then mix in the parsley, pepper, salt and garlic. Combine this with the egg and oats mixture.

Coat an egg skillet with nonstick spray, then pour ½ tsp olive oil into it. Heat skillet to medium, then add ½ cup of the mixture to the skillet and spread it with the back of a spoon to create a 6" pancake. Cook for three to four minutes before flipping it and cook the other side for three to four minutes or until golden brown. Repeat process, each time adding one tsp of oil first -- makes six pancakes.

The first two days, make the egg muffins and have two to three for breakfast with a protein shake. No milk with your eggs or in the protein shakes. Day 3 you can eat the protein pancakes for breakfast.

Make a batch of them and you can easily warm them up in the microwave. The only liquids allowed are water and unsweetened green tea.

Lunch

Allow yourself some protein. Grab a salad with adding eggs and/or grilled chicken. Do not use thick dressing like Thousand Island or Ranch. Use a light dressing or none at all. Have the salad only for lunch. Feel free to add flax seed oil in the salad.

3 hours later have a protein shake, mixed with water or almond milk (remember to avoid protein shakes with artificial sweeteners).

<u>Dinner</u>

Have protein with green vegetables. This means lean chicken, beef, or fish with broccoli, spinach, or peppers. No breads or processed carbs. Take at least two grams of fish oil at bed.

This is the only time I will ask that you lower your caloric intake. You want your body to cleanse and operate more efficiently. By not overloading your system, your body can heal and repair and start becoming a fat burning machine. Try the 2–1 approach. If you like the simple Quik Start breakfast, then do it for a few weeks.

Just do YOUR best. Remember, health restoration and weight loss is not a straight line. It curves, bends, reverses, and comes back around. Just keep moving forward. As Tony Little, the infomercial ponytail guy said, " YOU CAN DO IT!"

Chapter 14

Tips, Strategies and Stuff

If you Google weight loss, you will have more hits, links, blogs, and websites that you could read in a year. I will go ahead and summarize some of my favorite tips and bullet points. I may comment on whether I agree or disagree with some of these common points.

From an article at <u>USAToday.com</u>, I found "Weight loss tips -- 25 ways to lose weight and keep it off." The article says more than half of Americans want to lose weight. Almost all of them say they are trying to improve at least one aspect of their eating habits. The survey showed nearly 9 in 10 are trying to eat more fruits and veggies this survey showed. Of course these kinds of changes are easier said than done. This was from a study done by the International Food Information Council Foundation.

From the article, let us look at some of these weight loss tips:

1. <u>Set a realistic weight loss goal</u>. I would comment on that and say set smaller goals and one large goal. Again, if you shoot for the stars and only hit the moon, you have done well.
2. <u>Keep track of what you consume</u>. This would be a food diary or food log. When you write things down, you are more aware of what you are doing. You will also be more successful. This has been proven time and time again.
3. <u>Motivate yourself</u>. There are many ways of doing that. Find a picture of a person in a bathing suit, a pair of jeans, or an outfit that you would like to get. Put your picture or your face on that person's body. Heck, go out and buy that pair of jeans one size too small that you will fit into.

4. Enlist the help of family and friends. You can both help each other. When one is feeling little weaker, the other one can help you stay on track.

5. Move it to lose it. It is a good idea to remove yourself as far away as possible from a sedentary lifestyle. It is important that you do something on a regular basis. The point of the title of my book is to talk about how people fail. When the New Year's comes around, everybody starts adding exercise and gym memberships to their lifestyle that was not previously there. Without changing nutrition, you are going to tire yourself out and pretty much waste your efforts. People fail with their New Year's resolutions when it comes to weight lost because they do not make the lifestyle modifications that are necessary to change their physique. I see so many people go to the gym and walk on a treadmill for 30 minutes, then they pick up Subway with a Diet Coke and think they are obtaining a healthy body -- not true.

6. Pay attention to portions. I mean does anybody on this planet need a Big Gulp? Do we need to supersize our meals? Start creating smaller portions when you eat. Make a fist, and that is a good start of estimating the size and portion of protein you should eat.

7. Clean out your refrigerator. I believe this is self-explanatory. I have parents telling me they cannot get their kids to stop drinking so much soda. If you have it in the house, it is probably going to be difficult. If you do not buy it, they will not drink it. So clean up your food supplies.

8. Create a dinner deck. It is a list of foods that you can make. I would change that to say just be prepared. If you fail to plan, you are planning to fail. On Sundays I am prepared for all of my meals for the week.

9. Avoid hunger. You should be able to have healthy snacks throughout the day. Your meals should be frequent, about every three or four hours. I will say that there are times that we discussed doing cleanses or a controlled fast. But, as a general rule, you should constantly be grazing throughout the day. During times of lower caloric

intake, if you provide yourself with an adequate amount of water, that should help you from feeling hungry.

10. <u>Cut out liquid calories</u>. I think I discussed this enough in my book, if you are serious about becoming healthier and losing weight, then water should be the only liquid you are consuming, with the exception of green tea. Remember, "it's not what you do all the time, but what you do most the time that matters". Six meals per day, seven days a week, equals 42 meals. If you cheat 10% of the time, that is four cheat meals per week. That is plenty to keep your body happy and still be healthy.

11. <u>Pace don't race</u>. Eat slowly. There is a rule that you are supposed to chew each bite 25 times. Of course, I find that nearly impossible. But the point is to take your time when you are eating. Slow down and chew your food with smaller bites. Put your fork down between each bite. Take a breath, and take a sip of water. This will not only help with weight loss, but it prevents that insulin spike that we talked about, and also allows you to enjoy your meal.

12. <u>Hydrate before meals</u>. Having an eight-ounce glass of water before you eat, can make you feel fuller. Have another one at the end of the meal, and it will help as well.

13. <u>After eight is too late</u>. It is a nice motto to say that anything you consume after 8pm should only be a healthy snack.

14. <u>Treat yourself occasionally</u>. As I mentioned before, if 10% of your weekly meals are cheat meals, or I prefer to use a term reward, then you should still be able to enjoy everything that you love. I promise you, as you start changing your body and your mindset, these foods that you think you crave so much will be wanted far and few in between. What happens when you start losing weight, feeling better, and having more energy is that you get greedy. It happens every time. People start and lose 5 or 10 pounds, and then they want to go for 15 pounds.

15. <u>Eat without pigging out</u>. This goes with one the examples from above. Do not eat so fast and do not eat too many large quantities. This will create an insulin response, your

body will spike its blood sugar, and you go to fat <u>storage</u> mode versus fat <u>burning</u> mode. Just slow down, and, instead of living to eat, eat to live.

16. <u>Get plenty of sleep</u>. I have a whole chapter devoted to this. Sleep is very important to your health, well-being and, of course, weight loss.

17. <u>Eat at the table</u>. Do not eat in front of the TV or eat while you are in your car. Entertainment will distract you and will cause you to consume more food. You should also downsize your plates when preparing meals. The smaller the plate, the less room there is to pile on.

If you allow yourself to have a cheat meal or reward meal, enjoy it. Do not beat yourself up for it, you have earned it, you deserve it or frankly you just wanted it. The rule is your next meal must be healthy. So, therefore, you cannot have fast food for lunch and then say well I messed up so, therefore, I will have pizza for dinner. Make sure the next meal is healthy.

Just remember this, life, just like weight loss, or any other goal you create, is the journey, not the destination. Enjoy the ride.

Now, here are 25 healthy muscle-building foods that you can consume. I received this list from <u>naturalnews.com</u>.

1. Water
2. Whey protein
3. Whey protein powder
4. Free-range organic eggs
5. Raw milk. Now I have discussed to avoid milk. The only type of milk I would recommend is if you found a farm co-op and consumed unpasteurized milk from grass fed animals.
6. Bison: It is higher in protein than beef.
7. Free-range organic chicken breasts.
8. Grass-fed organic beef.
9. Fish: While salmon and tilapia are among the best. Try to avoid tuna due to the high mercury levels.
10. Turkey: A very lean protein source.
11. Nuts: Walnuts and almonds are the best.
12. Oysters: Great for naturally boosting testosterone levels.

13. Beans. A very slow digesting carb, high in zinc and fiber.
14. Oats.
15. Natural peanut butter: Higher healthy fats and protein, while low in carbohydrates.
16. Cottage cheese: Very low in sugar and high in protein.
17. Yogurt: Greek yogurt is the best.
18. Bananas: A potassium and vitamin-rich food.
19. Avocados: Very rich in unsaturated fatty acids.
20. Healthy oils: Extra virgin olive oil, coconut oil, walnut oil, hemp oil and flaxseed oil.
21. Spinach and other green leafy vegetables.
22. Broccoli: A super food and vegetable. Others include tomatoes, kale, cauliflower and bok choy.
23. Berries: High in antioxidants and many other vitamins necessary for muscle growth.
24. Quinoa and brown rice. Both are rich in B vitamins and slow digesting.
25. Apples and other fruit: High in fiber, which cleanses the system and allows for better nutrient absorption.

So, two weeks ago at my office, I asked five women to put together a food diary for me. I told them I wanted them to write down everything that they eat for breakfast, lunch, dinner, and snacks, to include any liquids and/or medications that they put in their bodies. Two weeks later and all five have failed to do their homework. So why am I sharing this information with you? The reason I share this is because this is up to YOU. If you are waiting for the magic pill or the magic food that you are going to consume and have that perfect body, then you need to wake up from your dream. I tell my patients all the time, this is YOUR health. It is not mine, it is not your spouses, it is not your children's, it is YOURS!

I purchased a book recently on weight loss because it had a catchy one-word title written by a doctor. The title of the book should have been changed to "dread". In my opinion, it is filled with so much outdated information. If you want to lose weight on a scale, then go to the local high school and talk to the wrestling coach and how you can lose a whole bunch of pounds on the scale. I do not want you to do that. I want you to be healthy. That is why the name of my Chiropractic website for my practice is called becomehealthier.com.

Anybody can drop pounds on a scale. However, it is the conversion of more lean muscle and the removal of excess body fat that is going to save your life. Not only will it save your life, it will extend the quality of your life. I do not want to you to drink one diet soda a day and think that is okay. Frankly it is not okay. You must make a few sacrifices in your life for the greater good of your health.

This is a summary from one of my favorite sources of fitness information, charlespoliquin.com. The article is called the "Top Ten Pitfalls to Weight Loss".

They are the following:
1. Do not eliminate fat. You need fat in your diet.
2. Get a balance fat intake.
3. Get rid of stress and lower cortisol levels.
4. Fix your gut by taking a PRO-biotic.
5. Support digestion with an HCL supplement.
6. Eat breakfast with protein in it. No cereal allowed.
7. Take a very cautious approach with the science and health media
    (mainstream or popular beliefs may be outdated research).
8. Do not trust the RDA and U.S. nutritional labels (very antiquated).
9. Focus on detoxification.
10. Do not forget to be active and strength train.

When you have the time, please go to that website and search for that article. It is filled with more detailed information. It is well worth your time to also learn the reasons WHY those 10 pitfalls will disallow you to never reach your health goals.

The last tidbit of information that I want to give you and explore more on your own is the subject of intermittent fasting. This can be an entire chapter on its own, but for my goal for you, I feel you should read about it and try it on occasion and see how YOUR body responds.

Intermittent fasting is just how it sounds. It is periods of planned and controlled breaks of consuming any type of food. If you take the time and go to Mercola.com and search at his website, you will find a lot of information on this subject. I personally have done intermittent fasting and find it incredibly beneficial to my health. Think of it like a machine at a factory. Eventually the machine needs a break and needs to cool down. Keep pushing a machine without a rest period or even routine maintenance and it will not perform as well as it should have in the future. Your body needs a break. It needs time to "cool down", heal and repair and frankly re-set.

The following is a summary from a recent article and video at Dr. Mercola's website on intermittent fasting:

- It has long been known that calorie restriction can increase the lifespan of certain animals. More recent research suggests that intermittent fasting can provide the same health benefits as constant calorie restriction, which may be helpful for those who cannot successfully reduce their everyday calorie intake.
- "Under-nutrition without mal-nutrition" is the only experimental approach that consistently improves survival in animals with cancer, and extends overall lifespan by about 30 percent.
- Both intermittent fasting and continuous calorie restriction have been shown to produce weight loss and improve metabolic disease risk markers. However, intermittent fasting tends to be slightly more effective for reducing insulin resistance.
- Besides turning you into an efficient fat burner, intermittent fasting can also boost your level of HGH production by as much as 1,200% for women and 2,000% for men.
- Intermittent fasting can improve brain function by boosting production of the protein BDNF, which activates brain stem cells to convert into new neurons and triggers other chemicals that promote neural health. This protein also protects your brain cells from changes associated with Alzheimer's and Parkinson's disease, and helps protect your neuro-muscular system from degradation.

Please experiment with this process during your journey to better health. I truly believe that this can help regulate your internal chemistry while giving your body a break. People cannot keep pushing their bodies to overwork from the poor food choices without any consequences.

This is not something that you will do everyday or even every week. This is also something that you do not do for a full day or multiple days. This may be something that a few times per month you perform intermittent fasting to allow your body to "catch-up" and self-regulate.

There are numerous variations of intermittent fasting. Daily fasting, several days each week or just a few times per month. Give it a try. As long as you mix it up when you do it, your body will not go to starvation mode. For me, 2-3 times each month seems to be appropriate. Of course this is also with good eating habits. We are not going to have a bunch of pizza and wings then fast to make up for that meal. Health is a journey, not a destination.

Chapter 15

Conclusion

Well, I really hope you enjoyed the information I provided in this book. This is not just a weight loss book, it is a health book. If there is information in this book that you already knew, then ask yourself, how hard have you tried to apply it. I believe it was in my Introduction that I said, "knowledge is not necessarily power, it is the <u>application</u> of knowledge that is power".

I have mentioned numerous times that I have a full-time practice, a full-time life, three young kids, all in sports, which can make life challenging at times. Nobody said losing weight or becoming healthier is easy. At times it is definitely a struggle. However, the more that you will apply the knowledge in this book, the greater your chances are for optimal health.

Optimal health can also mean optimal weight. However, optimal weight does not necessarily mean optimal health. I can give plenty of examples of chain smokers, who drank way too much alcohol, that are really thin. Does that mean they are also healthy? The information in this book all comes down to the basics. It is the fundamental knowledge of physiology, anatomy, and nutrition.

There are so many people that are either born with disabilities or have serious health issues that they are forced to deal with it. Let me give you an example. I took all three of my boys up to our local YMCA to get some exercise. One of my children decided that he was a little too tired to run around in the gym. One of his classmates was there, but he was in a wheelchair. This young boy in a wheelchair was playing basketball and having a great old time. I would bet, without talking to this child, that he would give anything to be able to run around. I told my son that you cannot take your health for granted. You have the ability to run around and be healthy, while another child does not have that opportunity.

Do not misunderstand what I am trying to tell you. We all get tired and we all get sore. <u>But what I am trying convey to you is that health is a choice and do not ever take it for granted</u>. Sometimes, when it is gone, it is gone. I see new patients every day at my office that have let their health deteriorate to the point of a less than desirable lifestyle.

I fully understand that many of you may not radically alter your lifestyle over the course of reading this book. But, I would be happy if many of you e-mailed me and said you started doing things that you learned, and that this book has made a difference for you. And from that difference of feeling better and having a little bit more energy, you decided to try a 10K. From the 10K, you have turned that into weight training, and you have influenced other people in your family to live a healthier lifestyle.

I said this in my book, and I frequently tell this to my patients: If you had a choice between chiropractic care, exercising, or proper nutrition, which will give you the biggest bang for your buck. The answer <u>is always</u> nutrition. If nutrition was a spot on a Vegas gambling table, by placing your chips on nutrition, you are going to win most of the time.

As I am writing this Conclusion, I spent the previous weekend at my oldest son's travel baseball tournament. I also just came home from my middle son's kid's cross fit exercise class. What I see happening with younger children and kids today, is the same problem that we have as adults. The problem that we all have is poor nutrition. I saw two overweight kids being told to push themselves by their overweight father sucking down Gatorade. All of them were drinking Gatorade. And after the baseball game, what are most kids given by their parents? Gatorade and a bag of chips. Most kids can get away with this kind of eating, because their insulin and blood sugar (things I have talked about) are not that poorly regulated. Continue with that lifestyle and choices, they will suffer obesity, cancer, and heart disease just like anyone else.

Being a doctor for years, I have seen people destroy their health very quickly. I have also seen people restore their health in a short period of time. Sadly, I think it is harder to restore your health, than it is to destroy it. <u>You have the ability inside of you to become healthier – DO IT!</u>

There are many shortcuts and fads that people try, as I discussed. During the time frame that I wrote this book, another fad has come out. The new buzzword right now is raspberry ketones. Yes, because THAT is the secret to weight loss and better health. Please, you do not need a magic formula or a certain potion or lotion. What you need is sound nutritional discipline.

I know the title of my book is *No Gym Go Slim*. I even talk about specific ways to maximize your exercise routines should you choose to add that. But the point that I need to repeat, and then I need to repeat some more, is the fact <u>it is all nutrition</u>. Some of my friends are telling me that their kids are getting chubby. They need to get their kids doing something. My advice to them is stop buying your kids soda. Stop feeding them so much processed food. When you do those things, THEN if you add exercise or activity, it will just further the process. You should know that fat cannot be released in the body if you continue to add toxins. Remove the toxins and you will remove the fat. Green veggies, chia seeds, aloe vera, parsley and cilantro absorb toxins in your body and help to eliminate them.

I wrote this book to help people. This is my first official book. I have decided that I am going to write several others. I am going to write a book about how important proper nutrition along with other health-related topics are essential to the healthy development and proper growth of children. People always mess it up. We get in our own way.

I am not trying to preach, I simply want to teach. My three kids, ages 11, 9, and 5 have never been to a pediatrician, nor have they ever had a medication. That does not mean because I am a Chiropractor that I am anti-medicine or anti-surgery. I do not say that to sound all-cool and boast about my kids. I say that because, for the most part, my kids eat really well and have been receiving Chiropractic care since the day they were born. Their bodies function normal and at an optimal level.

The younger we are, the faster we heal, and kids have such a strong immune system. Imagine that now as we get older, it takes a little longer for the body to heal or our immune system is a little bit less than what could be. Because of this, as you get older you need to do more and more to protect your health. It all starts with the information in this book.

Recently I fell and injured my ribs. There were no apparent fractures or breaks, which was great. I just had a lot of pain. Mostly I would call this a soft tissue injury. Soft tissues take six to eight weeks to heal. The reason I bring this up is the fact that with proper nutrition, your body will function better but can actually heal a bit faster. So I made sure to do everything extra with my nutrition that I could so that I can heal faster.

So, do me a favor. Do your best. Compete with you. Lead by example. Frankly, at the end of the day it does not matter about your husband or wife or kids or family or friends or neighbors, it all starts with you. You can do it. Do not tell me you can't. I know you can. How can I say that without knowing you? After almost two decades in health-care and meeting and talking with patients and instructors and reading, I know different than most when it comes to becoming healthier.

I still tell my patients that there are only two require-ments to go to the Chiropractor. You have to have a spine and you have to be alive.

We have to separate science from science fiction in this country. The FDA and the creators of the antiquated food pyramid would frown upon a diet that consisted of no grains and no dairy. I, of course, disagree with most of what the FDA does and says.

Lastly, you have to apply these principles of nutrition, which will allow you to lose weight and truly be healthy.

You have now completed this book. The choice is now yours. Do you want to be a typical American that comes with all the typical diseases, or are you ready to lose weight, be lean and have an abundance of energy. The choice is truly yours. When your WHY is big enough, you will figure out the HOW. When you make the conscious choice to become healthier, you will start saying things internally, and your body will thank you for saying things like "every day in every way I am getting healthier and healthier".

I hope you find my information useful and helpful. The word doctor means teacher. I have attempted to give you the best amount of information that I could provide and hope that it will, at least, give you the opportunity to make better choices. Just remember that health is cumulative. Most people with poor health did not suffer from an accident or trauma. Most people with poor health have mismanaged their bodies for a long time. I wish you nothing but the best in your pursuits of optimal health, wellness, and well being.

I have no preconceived thoughts, goals, or wishes for the number of people that may read this book. I hope that people read this book and then apply the information to their lives. I hope you read the book and give it to someone else who needs. Helping others will also help you achieve your goals.

The website for this book is the name of the book. It is nogymgoslim.com. I hope that many of you will check out the website, and allow me to post testimonials. There you will find my list of vitamins, minerals, supplements, and other items, that I recommended throughout this book, that are required for optimal health and weight loss. I would also like to be able to respond to your e-mails whenever possible, so that I can further assist you on your journey to truly becoming healthier and living a life with quality. You do not have to be great to start, you have to start to be great!

I wish you nothing but the best for you and your family. I am sincerely grateful for you taking the time to read my book. Be well for today and tomorrow.

Sincerely,

Dr. Richard L. Sheppard